Tackling NHS Jargon

Getting the message across

Sarah Carr

Writer and Editor
Carr Consultancy
Warrington

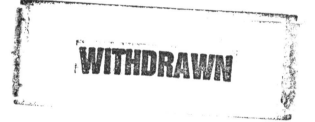
Radcliffe Medical Press

Radcliffe Medical Press Ltd
18 Marcham Road
Abingdon
Oxon OX14 1AA
United Kingdom

www.radcliffe-oxford.com
The Radcliffe Medical Press electronic catalogue and online ordering facility.
Direct sales to anywhere in the world.

British Library Cataloguing in Publication Data

A catalogue record for this book is available from the British Library.

ISBN 1 85775 428 X

Typeset by Acorn Bookwork, Salisbury, Wilts
Printed and bound by TJ International Ltd, Padstow, Cornwall

CONTENTS

Preface   v

User's guide   vii

Part One   NHS jargon   1

1   Recognising and categorising NHS jargon   3

Part Two   Jargon and the organisation   15

2   Encouraging a plain-communicating organisation   17
3   Describing benefits to staff   23
4   Convincing enough of the right people   31
5   Involving people in linking research to practice   41

Part Three   Plain language guidelines   49

6   Planning your plain document   51
7   Writing plainly   61
8   Tackling NHS jargon   75
9   Testing and revising your plain document   91
10   Communicating in speech and other special circumstances   103

Part Four   Aids to NHS jargon busting   113

Examples of NHS buzz words, with plain English translations   115

Examples of NHS gobbledegook, with plain English translations   121

Examples of NHS technical jargon, with plain English explanations   135

Example of a short style guide   153

Index   159

PREFACE

Roger has ... a speech problem. One which prevents him from speaking intelligently in the presence of his business peers. Here is something Roger said recently to a colleague: 'The client has an overly high expectation, market penetration-wise'.

What does it mean? Nothing, I'm afraid. Roger is talking nonsense. But did his colleague turn round and say: 'What is that meant to mean, for heaven's sake?' No, I'm afraid he did not. What he said was: 'Well, when you're in a customer-focused situation, you need more product awareness than their sort of low-profile image is going to generate'.

Yes, when Roger talks nonsense, his colleague talks nonsense back at him.[1]

I must admit that my interest in jargon started as a benign (and often entertaining) form of people watching, in my six years as an NHS manager. Listening to the language around me, I was often struck by how like Roger's and his colleague's it was – obscure yet contagious.

But although jargon is often treated in a light hearted manner, it is not really a laughing matter. Used properly, jargon can be fine and good. But it can also seriously damage your communications, wasting time and money, harming public, patient and staff relations, and dulling your thinking.

In my work since, writing and editing documents for the NHS, I have realised how few people know about the basic guidelines for communicating plainly. In an NHS highly concerned with evidence-based clinical practice, and increasingly interested in evidence-based management, evidence-based communication has so far not caught on. This book aims to help remedy this situation.

As with other human foibles, using jargon is something we like to think others do and we don't. But no one is perfect, and you will no doubt find places in this book where I could have got my message across more plainly.

If you do, please let me know. I would also be pleased to hear any other of your comments and suggestions, which I could use in my work with the NHS, and perhaps incorporate in a second edition of this book.

Finally, I would like to thank Tim Albert, Chris Divers, Chris Griffiths, Paula Moran and Liz Walker, for all their different forms of help, encouragement and support.

Sarah Carr
August 2001
secarr@carrconsult.u-net.com

REFERENCE

1   Kington M (1992) Severe case of sentence overload. *The Independent.* **13 April**: 18.

USER'S GUIDE

STRUCTURE

Parts One, Two and Three take you through the key stages in tackling NHS jargon, step by step. These are important for establishing a framework, and defining various terms used and developed in the rest of the book. I recommend that you read through the whole of these parts, in order.

Part Four is rather different; it provides lists of NHS jargon with suggested alternatives or explanations. I intend these to be used in two ways:

- as 'ready-made' alternatives to, and explanations for, some common NHS jargon, in plain English, for you to slot into your own communications – so saving you time and effort
- as examples of how to tackle NHS jargon, so providing further illustration of the guidelines given in Part Three.

A flowchart repeated at the beginning of each part of the book summarises the key stages in tackling NHS jargon. It also shows where to find each stage in the book, and which stage(s) will be covered in that part.

DEFINITIONS

For simplicity and clarity, I use the terms:

- '**NHS communicators**' to refer to all members of the book's target audience – not just communications managers and public relations officers, but all other staff who write and speak for or about the NHS. This includes NHS managers, clinicians with management responsibility (from the full range of health professions), non-executive directors and community health council officers

- **'communications'** to mean all forms of language – written (either on paper or electronically, as on a website) and spoken (whether planned, for example a speech, video commentary or press statement, or spontaneous)
- **'document'** or **'text'** for written language only, whether a short piece intended for just one person (for example an email or letter), a longer document for a big audience (such as an annual report) or anything in between.

EXAMPLES

All my examples of jargon-ridden language are from real NHS management communications aimed at the public and other audiences who are likely to find jargon difficult to understand. Most examples are from written communications – mainly because sitting in meetings jotting down examples of jargon-ridden utterances would not do much for business! Some examples are from documents I wrote before I learned about the guidelines. In all examples, I have made only minor changes to protect the authors' and organisations' anonymity, and to add enough context to ensure the extracts make sense.

My rewrites (of both individual words and phrases, and larger pieces of language) are certainly not the only possible solutions. Nor are they necessarily the best ones, and you may well think of clearer or more accurate alternatives. If you do, please tell me.

To Chris Divers

For standing together, but not too near together:

'For the pillars of the temple stand apart,
and the oak tree and cypress grow not in each other's shadow.'

NHS JARGON

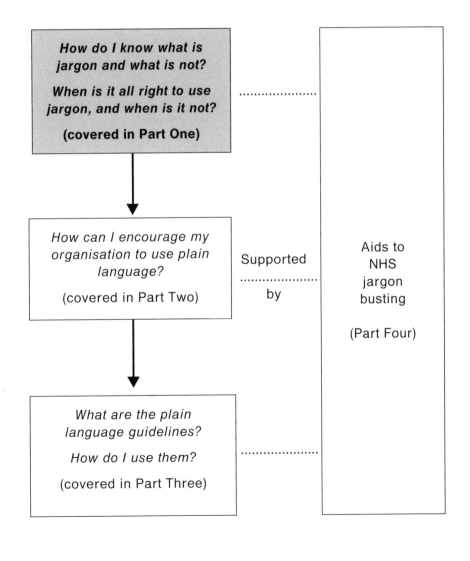

How do I know what is jargon and what is not?

When is it all right to use jargon, and when is it not?

(covered in Part One)

How can I encourage my organisation to use plain language?

(covered in Part Two)

What are the plain language guidelines?

How do I use them?

(covered in Part Three)

Supported
by

Aids to
NHS
jargon
busting

(Part Four)

CHAPTER 1

RECOGNISING AND CATEGORISING NHS JARGON

'Management-speak and gobbledegook are still rife in NHS documents. Poor communications still baffle patients and waste huge amounts of taxpayers' money.'[1]

Chrissie Maher, Founder-Director, Plain English Campaign

'Consult any National Health Service document nowadays and you will read of how "Government-wide agencies will provide effective services for all who benefit" and where "changes will need ownership of the guiding values ... a shared understanding within and across agencies and stakeholders".

...Little wonder, that with their [public sector managers'] eyes fixed firmly on creating their "cross-agency, cross-sector umbrellas", their projects should flounder in incompetence.'[2]

James Le Fanu, general practitioner and medical columnist

'We held public meetings fronted by GPs... At each meeting, three major problems were identified: communication, communication and communication. "You don't use our language." "You don't answer our questions." "You don't give us information in the right way." These same criticisms are made time and again in other surveys, in reviews and in public and internal inquiries. They were made after Hillsborough, after Dunblane, after the Piper Alpha disaster. They have been made in dozens of inquiries into shortcomings in systems, from health to education to sport.'[3]

    Hilary Spiers, Head of Communications, Cambridgeshire Health Authority

No one has anything good to say about NHS jargon. Members of the public complain it makes NHS communications hard to understand. NHS workers not involved in management find it confusing and alienating. Managers in partner organisations struggle to understand it. And those new to NHS management (such as management trainees, clinicians gaining management responsibility and new non-executive members) take time to learn it.

    But what exactly is jargon? Is it just one thing, or several? And is it always such a bad thing?

TYPES OF JARGON

The word 'jargon' comes from an old French word meaning 'the twittering and chattering of birds'. It came into English in the fourteenth century, when its meaning was extended to include 'meaningless talk' or 'gibberish'.

    The Longman Dictionary of Business English defines jargon as:

'(1) language, written or spoken, that is difficult or impossible for an ordinary person to understand because it is full of words known only to specialists

(2) language that uses words that are unnecessarily long and is badly put together.'[4]

Many linguists believe that the word 'jargon' would be best reserved for the first of the two definitions above. Some people also refer to this as 'technical jargon' or 'shop talk'.

    There have been many suggestions for words to describe the second type of jargon. The most popular today is probably 'gobbledegook', originally an American word thought to echo the sound of turkeys. Alternatives used over the years include 'bafflegab', 'bureaucratese', 'officialese', 'doublespeak', 'stripetrouser' (a lovely term invented by George Orwell) and 'FOG' (frequency of gobbledegook).

    A third type of jargon – buzz words and phrases – is also rife in the NHS. This fashionable jargon varies between areas of work, but is similar across public and private sector management.

    This book uses the terms '**technical jargon**', '**gobbledegook**' and '**buzz**

words' to differentiate these three main types of jargon – and '**jargon**' as a generic word to cover all of them. (If you read other work on jargon, remember that other writers may use these terms with slightly different meanings.)

CATEGORISING JARGON

It is important for NHS communicators to be able to:

- recognise jargon (so you can be aware when you or others are using it)
- understand how each of the three types of jargon – technical jargon, gobbledegook and buzz words – behaves (so you will know when to be watchful for each)
- differentiate between the three types of jargon (since there are different ways of tackling each).

TECHNICAL JARGON

Technical jargon is equally common in writing and in speech (both planned and spontaneous). In NHS management, it usually falls into one of the categories shown in Box 1.1.

Box 1.1: Categories of NHS technical jargon

- **Bodies** – names of specific bodies (e.g. 'Commission for Health Improvement', 'Health Development Agency'); or types of body (such as 'clinical directorate', 'primary care trust')
- **Staff groups** (for example 'nurse consultants', 'professionals allied to medicine', 'general dental practitioners')
- **Posts** (e.g. 'Caldicott guardian', 'complaints convenor')
- **Care types and services** (such as 'outpatient', 'daycase', 'community pharmacy', 'general medical services')
- **Documents** – names of specific documents (for example *Our Healthier Nation: a contract for health*', and '*The New NHS: modern, dependable*'); or types of document (such as 'White Paper', 'Green Paper', 'executive letter', 'health service circular')
- **Acts of Parliament** (e.g. 'the Mental Health Act 1983', 'the Disability Discrimination Act 1995')
- **Clinical specialties, conditions and treatments** referred to in management communications (for example 'ophthalmology', 'myocardial infarction', 'nicotine replacement therapy')

- **Initiatives, programmes and approaches** (such as 'Sure Start', 'Investors in People', 'integrated care pathways')
- **Concepts** (e.g. 'bed blocking', 'case-mix', 'clinical governance', 'earned autonomy')
- **Processes and activities** (such as 'benchmarking', 'commissioning', 'personal development planning')
- **Measures and standards** (for example 'standardised mortality ratio', 'chartermark', 'finished consultant episode', 'external financing limit')
- **Funds and budgets** – specific funds (e.g. 'the New Opportunities Fund'); or types of budget (such as 'non cash-limited')

In other words, words and phrases that fall into the category of technical jargon are official names for things. Although plain English experts recommend being sparing with capital letters at the beginning of words, technical jargon terms are the sort of words that many people feel should start with capitals. You would not find them in an ordinary dictionary. You can see more examples of this type of jargon in Part Four (in 'Examples of NHS technical jargon, with plain English explanations').

Technical jargon sometimes uses words that are in themselves ordinary, but which are used in a certain profession to mean something much more specific. For example, the word 'bed' is an everyday word, with an apparently straightforward and obvious meaning. But the Value-for-Money Unit of the NHS Directorate at the Welsh Office defines it specifically as:

'a device or arrangement that may be used to permit a patient to lie down when the need to do so is a consequence of the patient's condition rather than a need for active intervention such as examination, diagnostic investigation, manipulative treatment, obstetric delivery or transport.'[1]

Many pieces of technical jargon are often shortened to acronyms or abbreviations, particularly in speech. This makes it doubly difficult for the uninitiated audience to work out what is meant. (Acronyms are abbreviations that are pronounced as a word, for example 'NICE' [National Institute for Clinical Excellence]; abbreviations are pronounced as a series of letters, for example 'FCE' [finished consultant episode].)

GOBBLEDEGOOK

For most NHS communicators, true gobbledegook is a feature of written language only (or of spoken language that has been prepared in writing and then read out). It is perhaps the most common form of jargon, which may explain why plain language guidelines focus on written language.

Gobbledegook contains many:

- long and often unusual words, including foreign ones (especially Latin, for example 'ad hoc', 'inter alia', 'modus operandi', 'prima facie')
- abstract nouns (words describing intangible things as opposed to material objects), for example 'activity', 'process', 'assessment', 'approach'. These are often combined with other nouns and adjectives (words that describe nouns) into long 'noun phrases', for example 'an environment of an economy of scale service delivery, and interactive health-related scenarios'.

You will find gobbledegook words and phrases in an ordinary dictionary. In fact, people who use gobbledegook sound like they have swallowed one. You can see more examples of words that are common in gobbledegook in Part Four (see 'Examples of NHS gobbledegook, with plain English translations').

Unlike the other two types of jargon, however, gobbledegook does not just involve individual words. You can recognise it too by the overall style, which typically:

- includes many long sentences (of 25 words or more)
- has complex structures (both for individual sentences and the overall document)
- is impersonal in tone.

You do hear gobbledegook words and phrases in spoken language, especially among people whose work exposes them to documents written in gobbledegook, such as NHS communicators. Politicians are similarly afflicted (remember Sir Humphrey Appleby, of *Yes, Minister* and *Yes, Prime Minister* fame). However, the structural features described above make true gobbledegook rare in spontaneous speech. This is because, when talking, we have much less time to plan what we are going to say than when we write. It would be difficult to create such dense and complex language quickly enough to speak it spontaneously.

Box 1.2 contains two sentences that are typical examples of gobbledegook. Both are long (40 and 47 words). There are many words with three or more syllables (marked in bold) and many abstract nouns (underlined). Other words would probably be unfamiliar to many people, for example *delivered* (for the more familiar 'achieved') and *endorse* (for 'support'). The structure of the sentences is not straightforward. Both include complex

---

Box 1.2: Examples of gobbledegook

It was noted that cash from the **management** **underspend** has been **identified** to support the <u>plan</u> but there was <u>concern</u> that if there were no monies **available** in the <u>future</u>, **interest** would drop and the <u>plan</u> would not be **delivered**.
(from the minutes of a primary care group board meeting)

Directors are asked to note the current **position**, be aware that there are likely to be further **developments** in the **situation** in coming <u>months</u> and endorse the <u>action</u> taken so far to address the Authority's **paramount** <u>concern</u>, which is the <u>health</u> and <u>well being</u> of local **residents**.
(from a health authority board paper)

---

noun phrases (for example, 'action taken so far to address the Authority's paramount concern, which is the health and well being of local residents'). The tone of each example is detached.

BUZZ WORDS

In contrast to gobbledegook, buzz words are used mainly in spoken language, perhaps because they have a slightly informal feel. They generally change frequently and spread rapidly. Buzz words are fashionable in management circles, and there is a constant stream of new ones. For example, at the time of writing, many people are 'picking the low-hanging fruit first' (in other words – as I understand the phrase – starting with the easiest things). Buzz words are often made up of everyday, simple words (which you will find in an ordinary dictionary), but their combined meaning tends to be obscure (and cannot be found in a dictionary).

Sometimes old buzz words just disappear, and sometimes they become part of ordinary language. For example, you can now find some of the old chestnuts (such as 'ballpark', 'to hit the ground running', and 'window of opportunity') in an ordinary dictionary. Where they do join the everyday language, they are usually thought of as clichés, and may be used in parodies of stereotypical managers. For example, a trust chief executive on *Coronation Street* asks a grandfather whose new-born grandchild has just been snatched whether he is 'up to speed on developments'. You can see more examples of common NHS buzz words (new and old) in Part Four (see 'Examples of NHS buzz words, with plain English translations').

Whereas technical jargon is usually created by the profession that subsequently uses it, buzz words commonly come from the technical jargon of other areas of life (leisure as well as work related). For example, there is a strong presence of sporting jargon in management, such as 'team player', 'key player', 'arena', 'to row in the same direction', and 'to have the ball'.

The source of buzz words is often interesting in itself, as it reflects the kind of image that those using the buzz words are trying to convey. For example, sporting jargon carries images of teamwork, vitality, exertion and action. Note that NHS buzz words are more often drawn from team sports than from individual ones. This has been particularly true since the growth of partnership working.

Buzz words from other fields that carry a similar 'action' image are also popular in management, for example 'to be on board', 'to trawl', 'a driver for change', 'to parachute in', 'to get up to speed', 'to fast-track', 'to helicopter up' and 'movers and shakers'. It is no coincidence that management buzz words are often verbs that describe physical actions. This is in stark contrast to the prevalence of abstract nouns in gobbledegook.

MIXED JARGON TYPES

It is rare for a communication to contain just one type of jargon. For example, technical jargon often appears with buzz words in spoken language, and with gobbledegook in written language.

Similarly, words and phrases may belong to more than one type at the same time. For example, the words 'competence', 'concordat' and 'to facilitate', if used in a general sense, are gobbledegook. They could easily be replaced by simpler words like 'skill', 'deal' and 'to ease'. But if used with their more specific meaning (in the sense of skills that are part of National Vocational Qualifications, facilitating a discussion and the independent sector concordat), they are technical jargon.

THE VALUE OF JARGON

Jargon is often written off as a bad thing. But technical jargon is both necessary and useful for members of a profession or other group to communicate with each other. At its best, it acts as a kind of shorthand, allowing them to express specialist concepts concisely. It therefore improves the effectiveness of communication and saves time (and so money). For example, using the word 'bed' with the specific meaning given earlier in this chapter (as a much shorter version of the full definition) is both fine and sensible, so long as everyone talking about it is familiar with this meaning.

The problems only start when members of a profession inadvertently or otherwise use technical jargon in writing or speaking to people who are not familiar with it, without explaining what it means. This is easily done, as they are everyday terms to us, slipping off most of our tongues regularly. It is easy to get it wrong and forget that they will not be familiar to the audience. Ordinary words (such as 'bed'), used with a specific meaning that you do not make clear, are particularly dangerous, as a general audience would think they had understood but actually not have done.

However, it is not only perfectly acceptable, but also positively advantageous, to include technical jargon in communications for the public and other groups who are not familiar with it, so long as it is well explained. There are two main reasons for this:

- From a practical point of view, it is impossible for the writer/speaker to replace completely most of the words and phrases that fall into the category of technical jargon with plain English translations that are concise and accurate in meaning. Understanding this is the first step to being able to deal effectively with technical jargon, but a step that many people do not recognise. Much energy can be expended, time wasted and frustration built up in trying to think up the perfect short phrase to substitute for 'primary care' or 'clinical governance', when the truth is that one probably does not exist!
- From an ethical point of view, exposing the audience to the standard terms for NHS bodies, concepts and so on, as used throughout the NHS, can help them to understand more about the NHS. This, in turn, can empower them, for example to understand how the NHS works and to get more involved in its running. Members of the public – or whoever your target audience might be – accept that all professions have technical terms, and may in fact like to hear them – so long as they are explained properly.

For example, if several different NHS communicators all eliminated the term 'clinical governance' by replacing it with a plain English alternative, they would:

- probably end up with long-winded and complex sentences
- stop the audience from recognising the term 'clinical governance' if they subsequently came across it in other contexts
- prevent the audience from looking up more information about the term elsewhere
- probably all give slightly different explanations, so preventing the audience from realising they were all talking about the same thing
- risk making the audience feel they were not making an effort to keep them fully informed, and perhaps even sound patronising.

Table 1.1   Key characteristics of NHS jargon

	Type of NHS jargon		
	Technical jargon	*Gobbledegook*	*Buzz words*
Typical linguistic features	• Official names for things • Often spelt with capital letters • Commonly shortened to abbreviations or acronyms	• Long words • Abstract nouns • Latin words • Long-winded, complex and impersonal style	• Many verbs • Often derived from other fields, especially sports
Common in NHS writing?	Yes	Yes	To an extent
Common in NHS planned speech?	Yes	To an extent	To an extent
Common in NHS spontaneous speech?	Yes	Only words and phrases, not structures	Yes
Rate of change	Depends on rate of change of government policy for the NHS (so usually fairly fast!)	Slow	Fast
In an ordinary dictionary?	No	Yes	No
Relative length of plain English alternatives	Longer	Shorter	Varies
Effect on communication	Positive – if used with audience that understands it, or explained to audience that does not Negative – if used unexplained with audience that does not understand it	Negative	Negative

Take the analogy of patients going to see their GP. They want to be given a clear explanation of their diagnosis, in layperson's language, but they may well find it useful to be given the medical term too. They will then know if their diagnosis is the same as that of someone else they know, be able to look up more about it in a health book or on a health website, and feel that the doctor credited them with the ability and interest to hear and use the medical term. Chapter 8 describes ways of retaining NHS technical jargon, while explaining it in plain English.

Buzz words can be similarly useful as a type of shorthand, as their plain English translations are often longer. However, the big problem is that the meaning of buzz words is often obscure, even among colleagues. This means that a group of NHS communicators who think they know what is meant by a particular buzz word may in fact all be interpreting it differently. Even if the meaning of a buzz word has become more agreed (by joining the ordinary language and so being defined in a dictionary), it is likely to be clichéd. Therefore, if you want to be sure of communicating your message clearly, buzz words are best avoided.

Gobbledegook, meanwhile, can almost always be replaced by plain English alternatives that are less long-winded (and, again, clearer in meaning).

Table 1.1 summarises the key characteristics and value of technical jargon, gobbledegook and buzz words.

In the last row of Table 1.1, the shaded areas show those parts of NHS jargon use that have a negative impact on communication – and are therefore worth tackling. The unshaded area shows that part of jargon use that helps communication. In the rest of the book, these areas of jargon use will be referred to as 'negative jargon use' and 'positive jargon use' respectively. The choice of these terms is intended to show that:

- (in the case of technical jargon) it is the use of the jargon – as opposed to the jargon itself – that has a negative effect on communication
- the shaded areas of jargon use should be avoided only because they have a proven negative effect on communication, as Chapter 3 will show. (Value judgements on language and language use are all too rife.)

Communicating with the target audience in a way that its members can easily understand will be referred to simply as 'plain language'.

REFERENCES

1   Friend B (1998) Calling a bed a bed. *Health Service Journal.* **108** (5594): 31-3.
2   Le Fanu J (2001) Speaking words imperfect. *The Daily Telegraph.* **13 March**: 18.

3   Spiers H (1998) Clarity begins at home. *Health Service Journal.* **108** (5594): 28-30.

4   Adam JH (1982) *Longman Dictionary of Business English.* Longman, Harlow, p. 261.

Jargon and the Organisation

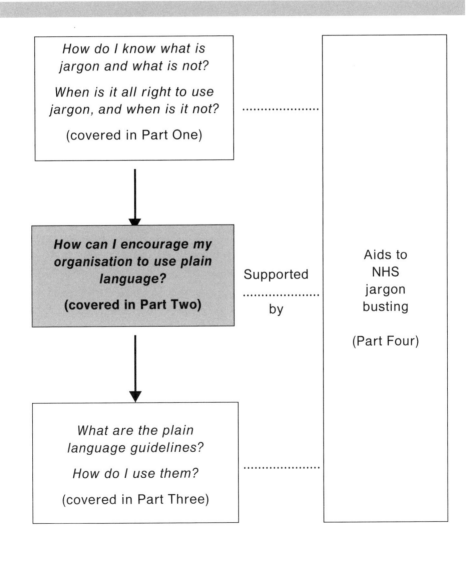

How do I know what is jargon and what is not?

When is it all right to use jargon, and when is it not?

(covered in Part One)

How can I encourage my organisation to use plain language?

(covered in Part Two)

What are the plain language guidelines?

How do I use them?

(covered in Part Three)

Supported by

Aids to NHS jargon busting

(Part Four)

CHAPTER 2

ENCOURAGING A PLAIN-COMMUNICATING ORGANISATION

So why develop skills in plain speaking and plain writing throughout the organisation? It might seem easier just to pay a consultant, or train a small number of NHS communicators, to write important communications in (or edit them into) plain English.

In fact, you may, at least in the early days (and perhaps always), choose to use external experts for major documents, for example annual reports. Even when your own communicators are sufficiently skilled in plain language, there are busy times when it is worth paying an extra pair of skilled hands to write a time-consuming document. And you may choose to train some staff to a higher level than others. But if you rely entirely on external experts, or a small group of staff, your organisation will be missing out on many benefits. These come from encouraging everyone to use plain language, in speech and writing, in both external and internal communications.

To bring about a plain-communicating organisation, NHS communicators must be aware of, and understand, the plain English guidelines (covered in Part Three). However, this is not enough to bring about lasting change. Preparing the ground is essential, particularly in terms of organisational culture and people's attitudes.

IMPLEMENTING PLAIN LANGUAGE

The process of introducing plain language is essentially the same as that of implementing any other evidence-based change in practice.

   You are almost certainly more experienced and skilled than I am at implementing change. This book does not therefore give you exhaustive instructions on how to introduce plain language to your NHS organisation. Instead, it aims to support your management skills by:

- providing evidence (research based where possible) that you can use to help implement plain language
- giving you practical hints on aspects of introducing change that may be peculiar to implementing plain language (based on my consultancy experience and other writers' advice).

These hints and evidence are organised into categories based on Wye and McClenahan's four essential factors in putting research evidence into practice (*see* Box 2.1). Wye and McClenahan derived these factors from an evaluation of the effectiveness of different approaches used by 15 project teams carrying out 17 projects funded by the North Thames Research & Development Directorate.[1]

Box 2.1: Essential factors in putting research evidence into practice

- Resources – of time, money and skills – need to be sufficient (covered in this chapter)
- The proposed change needs to offer benefits of real interest to staff who have to change (Chapter 3)
- Enough of the right people need to be on board [note the buzz words!] early enough (Chapter 4)
- The approach needs to be interactive (or, to avoid gobbledegook, involve people) and relate research clearly to practice (Chapter 5)

RESOURCES REQUIRED

To implement plain language in line with the principles and methods recommended in Chapters 3 to 5, you will need sufficient time, money and skills. Time and money are closely related, since the main investment required is in staff time.

   Finding time and money is never easy in the NHS. But if you can manage it, the initial costs will be more than compensated for by the time and money savings that will ensue. (These and other more qualitative benefits, which you should also weigh against the initial costs, are described in Chapter 3.) It is important to remember, however, that, as with many other changes, things do not happen overnight. The process of changing behaviour is inevitably a gradual one.

Once people have learned the new habit of communicating in plain language, doing so will take no longer – and may even take less time (though more thought and skill) – than communicating in the old, jargon-ridden style. It will become easier – and so quicker – all the time.

The other main element of financial cost will be that of acquiring or buying in the necessary skills. You will need three main types of skill or knowledge:

- skills in managing change. You should already have these in your organisation
- knowledge of the facts relating to plain language, for example its benefits, reasons for negative jargon use, objections to plain language, and responses to these objections. You can learn the facts you need to implement plain language by reading this book
- skills in understanding and applying (and in helping others to understand and apply) plain language guidelines. These may well be lacking, and are more difficult to acquire just from reading.

In short, although there are plain language consultants who will be only too happy to supply the first two types of skill, you almost certainly do not need their assistance. Look on them as an extra pair of (skilled) hands rather than a unique source of expert advice and knowledge – they may provide useful support if everyone in the organisation is pushed for time.

UK organisations providing training in the third type of skill include those listed in Box 2.2. (All tend to concentrate on written, as opposed to spoken, communication skills.) There may also be smaller, local organisations or individuals working in this field.

Box 2.2: Examples of organisations providing training in communication skills

Plain English Campaign	Telephone:	01663 744409
PO Box 3	Fax:	01663 747038
New Mills	Email:	info@plainenglish.co.uk
Stockport SK12 4QP	Website:	http://www.plainenglish.co.uk

Plain English Commission The Castle 29 Stoneheads Whaley Bridge High Peak SK23 7BB	Telephone: Fax: Email: Website:	01663 733177 01663 735135 cutts@clearest.co.uk **or** cutts@plainlanguage.demon. co.uk http://www.clearest.co.uk http://www.plainlanguage. demon.co.uk
The Word Centre 27 Norfolk Hill Sheffield S35 8QA	Telephone: Fax: Email: Website:	0114 257 1400 0114 257 1528 df@wordcentre.co.uk http://www.wordcentre.co.uk
Tim Albert Training Paper Mews Court 284 High Street Dorking Surrey RH4 1QT	Telephone: Fax: Email: Website:	01306 877993 01306 877929 tatraining@compuserve.com http://www.timalbert.co.uk

(The courses run by Tim Albert Training include plain English guidelines, in the broader context of effective writing processes.)

Various different types of training are available. Typical course types are listed in Table 2.1, together with their key features and typical costs.

In deciding which courses are going to be the most cost-effective, you need to consider how many people you need to train, and to what level. For example, you may have large numbers to train, or anticipate a long-term need for training (for example because of high staff turnover). In these cases, it would probably be more cost-effective to train your own trainers.

Organisations such as the Plain English Campaign, the Plain English Commission and the Word Centre commonly also provide other services. These include consultancy support, writing and editing services, kitemarking schemes and corporate membership (usually comprising regular newsletters and discounts on other services).

This chapter has already mentioned the possible uses of consultancy support, and writing and editing services. (Incidentally, there are also many freelances offering general writing and editing services. Do not assume that they are adept at plain language writing and editing; it is surprising how few know the plain English guidelines.) Chapter 9 covers kitemarking schemes. You may find that joining a corporate membership scheme saves you money if you plan to use one organisation a lot, and that it helps signal (both internally and externally) your commitment to plain language.

Table 2.1: Types of training provided

Type of training	Key features	Typical cost at time of writing (excluding VAT)
'Teach yourself' course	• Course to work through by yourself • Usually has no tutor support	Some available on websites, free of charge; others to order at minimal cost
Open course	• Provided in central locations • For mixed groups from different organisations	£100 to £350 per person for one-day course
In-house course	• Delivered at the venue of your choice • For a maximum of around 12 people from your organisation • Usually run over one or two days	£800 to £1200 per day (for whole group)
Individual coaching session	• Tailor-made training for one person or a small number of people from your organisation	Consultancy rates (typically £800 to £1200 per day)
Advanced course	• Designed to develop plain English skills at a higher level • Part-time over a period of months	£2700 per person per course
'Training the trainers' course	• Designed to develop your own in-house plain English trainers • Packs of materials for use in training often available to buy	Structure of charges varies between organisations, and depends on the particular needs of your organisation and the skills of the individuals involved

REFERENCE

1   Wye L and McClenahan J (2000) *Getting Better with Evidence: experiences of putting evidence into practice.* King's Fund Publishing, London.

CHAPTER 3

DESCRIBING BENEFITS TO STAFF

As with all other types of change, it is no use trying to impose plain language on staff who are not convinced of its merits. Most people have views on what is 'good' and what is 'bad' English, and many are quick to voice their own views and to try to impose them on others. But views alone, however sound and well-intentioned, are unlikely to convince people to use plain language. Fortunately, there is an increasing body of anecdotal and research evidence showing that plain language benefits both the writer/speaker (and employing organisation) and the reader/listener. This is useful as a starting point. You can significantly reinforce this with evidence that plain language improves things in your own organisation.

THE SOURCE OF PLAIN LANGUAGE EVIDENCE

Evidence of the benefits of plain language comes not only from the UK but also from many other countries, including Australia, Canada, New Zealand, South Africa, Sweden and the US. The facts that the plain language movement is geographically so widespread, and that many of these countries have government backing for plain language initiatives, should help convince cynics of the benefits of plain language. Box 3.1 gives examples of plain language activities from around the world.

Box 3.1: Activities of plain language movements around the world

- In the **UK**, the government issued a White Paper in 1982 requiring that all its departments eliminated forms wherever possible and simplified the rest[1]
- In **Europe**, the European Commission's translation department launched a 'Fight the FOG' campaign, aiming to encourage clear communication in English, French, German and Italian[2]
- In **Sweden**, the Ministry of Justice has a Division for Legal and Linguistic Draft Revision, which converts all draft statutes into plain language[3]
- In **South Africa**, the Ministry of Justice has started a drive to write laws and government forms in plain language[3]
- In the **US**, the federal rules of civil, criminal and appellate procedure are now drafted in plain language[3]
- In **Canada**, several federal agencies created a partnership to develop a process for drafting in plain language[3]
- In **Australia**, the Parliamentary Counsels of Queensland and of New South Wales have publicly endorsed drafting in plain language[3]
- In **New Zealand**, the Law Commission has endorsed a plainer style of legislative drafting[3]
- **You can find the website of the Plain Language International Network at http://www.plainlanguagenetwork.org. This contains links to plain language organisations in many countries.**

Evidence of the benefits of plain language is based mainly on written (rather than spoken) communications. Although studies comparing original and revised texts have shown that a wide range of document types are improved by the use of plain language, there is an emphasis on legal documents. Perhaps not surprisingly, the plain language movement is particularly well developed in the field of law.

There is a lot of evidence on the benefits of using plain language in designing forms. This is probably because forms aim to get a specific response from their target audience (that is, a correctly completed form), in contrast to other types of document that aim to provide information. The forms researched in plain language studies tend also to be those that people need to fill in if they want to gain some service or benefit from the producing organisation (as opposed to those that people fill in as a favour to the produc-ing organisation). It is therefore relatively straightforward to measure, for example, how many people have understood a form by, say, the proportion of returned forms that are correctly completed, and the number of people seeking clarification or complaining. Costs to the organisation of a badly worded form are also more obvious, since the organisation will be aware of having to spend time getting incorrectly completed forms amended and dealing with queries.

Although some of the evidence comes from other countries, and some may not focus on the type of documents that NHS communicators typically produce, there is no reason why it should not apply to their written and spoken language.

WHAT BENEFITS DO STAFF WANT?

Wye and McClenahan[4] found that staff were pleased to receive thanks or recognition for their part in implementing change. But this in itself was not enough to get them to change their behaviour. The benefits that motivated managers most to put evidence into clinical practice were:

- savings in NHS time and money
- improved patient care.

'Improved patient care' clearly relates to changes in clinical practice. Its equivalent in the implementation of plain language is improved public and patient relations, achieved through better communication. This is good both for those with NHS management responsibility, and for patients and the public. Plain language also has much to offer internal communications, leading to improved staff relations.

SAVINGS IN TIME AND MONEY

Communicating in plain language:

- saves time (and so money) for the producing organisation, by reducing complaints, questions and misunderstandings from the target audience. Box 3.2 shows examples of this
- saves time (and possibly money) for members of the target audience, by reducing the amount of time they have to spend digesting the communication, and clarifying any points they do not understand. If the target audience for a communication is internal (for example staff), then the savings to the organisation are twofold. The staff at whom the communication is aimed spend less time digesting it and raising queries; those who produce it spend less time dealing with such queries. *See* Box 3.3 for examples.

Box 3.2: Evidence of time and money savings for the organisation[1]

- Before the Royal Mail had its redirection form put into plain English, there was an 87% error rate when customers filled it in. The organisation was spending a lot of money dealing with complaints and reprocessing the incorrect forms. The new form reduced the error rate dramatically, leading to savings of £500 000 over the following nine months
- The UK Ministry of Defence revised its civilian travel claim form, cutting the error rate by 50%, and so the processing time by 15%. It saves £400 000 a year in staff time
- When British Telecom adopted a plain language approach to telephone bills, the number of customer complaints and enquiries fell by 25%
- In the US, the General Electric Company put a software manual into plain language. It found that business customers who used a previous version of the manual made about 125 more calls a month than those who used the revised version. The company estimates that it saves between $22 000 and $375 000 a year for each business customer using the new manual

---

Box 3.3: Evidence of time and money savings for the target audience[1]

- In a study for the UK Department of Health and Social Security, Coopers & Lybrand concluded that errors on its forms cost employers and members of the public around £675 million
- By revising its duty-free allowances form, the UK Department of Customs and Excise reduced the error rate from 55% to 3%, saving passengers 7500 hours each year
- The US company Federal Express revised its operations manuals, which explained company procedures to staff. Staff using the old manuals took an average of 5 minutes to find information, and found the correct answer only 53% of the time. With the new manuals, the average search time dropped to 3.6 minutes, and the success rate improved to 80%. The company estimated that the new manuals would save $400 000 in staff time in the first year alone
- In the US, naval officers read a business memo written either in plain language or in a bureaucratic style. Those reading the plain language version took 17 to 23% less time to read it and felt less need to reread it. Understanding also improved. It was estimated that if all documents used plain language, the Navy would save $250 to $350 million a year

Plain language may also reduce printing and postage costs, since documents written in plain language tend to be shorter.

IMPROVED PUBLIC, PATIENT AND STAFF RELATIONS

Members of the target audience (whether internal or external) are likely to be pleased that their time and money are being saved. In the case of public sector bodies, such as the NHS, those members of the target audience who care about the efficient use of public funds may also be pleased that the organisation is saving time and money.

Savings in time and money for both the organisation producing the communication and its target audience come about because:

- the audience can understand plain language better
- plain language is faster for them to read.

There is also evidence that people prefer plain language. Box 3.4 gives evidence of these advantages of plain language.

Box 3.4: Evidence of people understanding and liking plain language better, and reading it faster

- In the UK, a focus group comprising people with a wide range of backgrounds gave ratings for clarity to 'before' and 'after' examples prepared for a book on plain language. In general, the group preferred the plain language versions[5]
- Again in the UK, the Plain Language Commission tested the Clearer Timeshare Act (a law rewritten in plain English) on senior law students. Ninety per cent preferred the plain version to the real act. Understanding also improved, with 94% getting the correct answer to one key question when using the revised version, against only 48% with the original one[5]
- In a US study, readers of a medical consent form were able to answer an average of 2.36 out of 5 questions correctly on the original form. However, they could answer an average of 4.52 on the revised version, a 91% improvement. The average response time also improved from 2.65 to 1.64 minutes[3]
- Again in the US, a study of two versions of a medical leaflet on polio vaccine showed that reading time dropped from almost 14 to about 4.5 minutes with the plain language one. Understanding also

improved, and the proportion saying that the chances they would read the leaflet went up from 49% to 81%[1]
- A study of US jury instructions presented to jurors orally showed that plain language versions improved understanding from 45 to 59% – an improvement of 31%.[3] (This study is particularly interesting in that it demonstrates the value of plain language in speech)
- In a study of legislation by the Law Reform Commission of Victoria, Australia, lawyers and law students understood plain language versions of the legislation in a third to a half of the average time needed to understand the original versions[1]

These advantages of plain language make the target audience more likely:

- to read or listen to the communication fully and attentively in the first place
- to feel positive towards the producing organisation (as opposed to thinking it pompous, insincere or ineffective)
- to believe that the producing organisation is being open with them.

This leads to better relations with the target audience – be it the public, patients, staff, or any other internal or external audience – and a better response to the communication.

In commercial organisations, all this brings increased sales. Although purchasing decisions are rather more complex in the NHS, it could be argued that better relations with the public and patients give providers a better image in the eyes of those who commission services from them. The public may also be more likely to ask for a referral to a provider that has better public relations.

But selling services is not the only purpose of the NHS. There is an increasing emphasis on the importance of public and patient involvement, on staff participation, and working in partnership with other NHS and non-NHS organisations. Effective communication is vital to all these developments, and so has implications for NHS communicators' appraisals and ultimately career progression.

CLEARER THINKING

As well as savings in time and money, and improved public, patient and staff relations, plain language has the important and valuable benefit (again to both organisation and audience) of promoting clearer thinking.

There does not seem to be any hard evidence for this, perhaps because it would be difficult to test and prove scientifically. However, practical experience of using plain language has convinced me that this is true. This is backed up by eminent practitioners in the field of plain language and business communications. They say that using plain language does impose a mental discipline that forces writers and speakers to be clear in their own minds about what they are trying to say (*see* Box 3.5). This brings organisations the further benefit of clearer planning and policy making.

Box 3.5: Anecdotal evidence of plain language promoting clearer thinking

- 'My boss and mentor for many years, HT Parker of Roles & Parker, ... taught us that only when you write down, for public consumption, what the instigators think they want to say can you see clearly whether or not it works. You can point to the holes still to be filled, you can ask the questions still to be answered, you can pinpoint what makes sense and what does not. Thus the professional communicator plays a key role in formulating policy, as opposed to simply delivering it.'[6]

  John Makin, past President, British Association of Communicators in Business

- 'Writing in plain language almost always improves the content. By improving structure and style, you improve the substance.'[1]

  Professor Joseph Kimble, Professor, Thomas Cooley Law School, USA – an internationally renowned expert on, and advocate of, plain language

---

REFERENCES

1   Kimble J (1996–97) Writing for dollars, writing to please. *The Scribes Journal of Legal Writing.* **6**.

2   Tim Albert Training (2000) Eurofight for clear English. *Short Words.* **9**(1): 1.

3   Kimble J (1994–95) Answering the critics of plain language. *The Scribes Journal of Legal Writing.* **5**.

4   Wye L and McClenahan J (2000) *Getting Better with Evidence: experiences of putting evidence into practice.* King's Fund Publishing, London.

5   Cutts M (1999) *Plain English Guide: how to write clearly and communicate better.* Oxford University Press, Oxford.

6   Makin J (2000) Talking point. *CiB News.* **7**(April): 2.

CHAPTER 4

CONVINCING ENOUGH OF THE RIGHT PEOPLE

In an ideal world, knowing about the real benefits of plain language would be enough to convince people to abandon negative jargon use. But real life is not that simple, and people often have deep-rooted reasons for this use of jargon. They may also have objections to using plain language that are based on highly entrenched views. Understanding these barriers is an important first step towards convincing people that it is acceptable to use plain language.

Getting people to turn their back on these reasons and objections is bound to be difficult. This is a delicate area, our language use being, in many ways, an extension of our personality, background and experiences. The way we use language at work is also affected by the culture of the NHS as a whole, and of the individual organisation. Although there can be no easy answers, this chapter looks at some common barriers to plain language, and suggests various ways of overcoming them.

BARRIERS TO PLAIN LANGUAGE

INAPPROPRIATE ATTITUDES AND VALUES

Some writers claim that communicators use jargon negatively for various dishonourable reasons, relating to their attitudes and values. In particular, professionals are said to use jargon:

- to show off and sound better than they are in some respect. For example, they use it to sound cleverer than they are, so excluding the uninitiated, and claiming membership of an exclusive club. Similarly, cynics might say that paper-pushing 'administrators' (as they would no doubt call managers) use action-based buzz words to make it sound as if they are harder working and more effective than they really are
- because they are lazy. Using convenient, ready-made buzz words or hiding weak ideas in a lot of gobbledegook saves having to think too much about what they are really saying
- to deceive the audience by hiding the truth behind euphemistic or unfathomable language (hence the term 'doublespeak' as an alternative name for gobbledegook). Examples of such 'political' writing include 'diminution of existing core service provision' (service cuts) and 'right-sizing' (making staff cuts).

Some NHS communicators, being only human, no doubt succumb now and then to one or more of these uses of jargon, whether intentionally or otherwise. But they are in a minority.

Certainly, to communicate successfully in plain language, you must genuinely want to get your message across honestly and effectively. The modern plain language movement is founded on a determination to ensure fair treatment for the public, by getting rid of language that stops them understanding their rights. Many of those who work for the plain language cause today do so because they have an ideological commitment to communicating honestly with the public. The majority of NHS communicators will no doubt be at home with these values, which are in keeping with both the public service ethic and the government's commitment to increased public and patient participation.

PERCEPTIONS OF 'PROPER' ENGLISH

Among the more innocent reasons for negative jargon use in the NHS is the belief that plain English is not 'proper' English. People often think it is too simplistic and that it excuses 'sloppy' grammar.

English teachers from our youth may have much to answer for here. Traditionally, pupils were often rewarded for the use of long and unusual words and complex sentence structures. Even those who have, in later years, discovered the plain language guidelines, and who see the benefits of applying them, often find it hard to go against the deeply ingrained lessons of their pasts.

In fact, many of the 'rules' that our English teachers taught us are not to do with grammar at all, but with conventional usage. Examples include not using split infinitives (such as 'to boldly go'), and not starting a sentence with 'and' or 'but' or ending one with a preposition (e.g. 'in', 'on' or 'up'). The truth is that most language experts do not outlaw these things at all.

Yet this traditional style lives on in the language of many highly esteemed professions (including medicine). This may be partly because their members have often had a traditional education, and because the traditional academic style of writing (particularly in the sciences) is dry and jargon ridden. People therefore tend to associate jargon-ridden language with being (or at least appearing) educated and intelligent. They are concerned that if they use simple language, others will think they too are simple. They genuinely believe that a jargon-ridden style sounds more sophisticated and more elegant.

Box 4.1 sets out several possible responses to these viewpoints.

Box 4.1: Responses to the belief that plain English is not 'proper' English

- Plain English is definitely not about bad grammar and poor linguistic standards. It has a long and respectable history in writing on English style. For example, two classic books that are still widely used today, HW Fowler's *A Dictionary of Modern English Usage*[1] and Sir Ernest Gowers' *The Complete Plain Words*[2], were originally published in 1926 and 1954 respectively. Both of these advise writers to apply principles that are in keeping with today's plain English guidelines
- It is much more difficult to simplify than to complicate ideas and language. Those who can think clearly through what they want to say, and communicate this effectively to their target audience, are more skilled than those who wrap their ideas in a jargon-ridden style
- In the field of law, readers assume that lawyers who use plain English come from more prestigious firms.[3] And a research study asking industrial and academic scientists to rate two short pieces of scientific writing showed that three-quarters judged the writer of the plain version to be more competent as a scientist and to have a better organised mind[4]
- Plain language guidelines are not intended to apply to literary writing, which, unlike business communications, is not just about getting a factual message across to its audience. However, plain English is in fact the style of many eminent authors, including Kingsley Amis, Somerset Maugham, George Orwell, Jonathan Swift, Mark Twain and Keith Waterhouse. And no one would say that these writers are simple
- A clear and straightforward communication can be beautiful in its simplicity and efficiency. Certainly, you should feel proud of producing a communication that the target audience understands

PLAIN LANGUAGE SEEN AS SIMPLISTIC

Related to the perception that plain language is not 'proper' English is the concern that you cannot express complex ideas in plain language. This is one of the main objections of those lawyers who are against having legal documents in plain language. But those who have translated legal writing into plain English are convinced that it is perfectly possible to express complex concepts plainly. For example, Professor Joseph Kimble states:

> 'Of all the barriers to change – and to realising the benefits of plain language – none is greater than the myth that clarity has to be sacrificed for precision, especially with complex subjects. Don't believe it. The murkiness that plagues so much official and legal prose is usually generated by the writer, not the substance. It comes more from bad style than from the inherent difficulty of the subject. And that's when the need for "precision" becomes a lame excuse for lame writing.'[5]

Moreover, there has been no noticeable rise in litigation as a result of plain English materials emerging,[6] nor has any company that has issued a plain English insurance policy, pension contract or bank guarantee ever chosen to go back to a traditional legalistic wording.[4]

Other people – outside the field of law – who are well qualified to talk about effective communication also believe that you can express complex ideas in plain language. For example:

> 'The most straightforward propositions are typically obscured in a flurry of clauses, compounds and impersonal passive tenses. But in fact with a little thought – and self-restraint – even the most complex notions can be expressed simply.'
>
> Peter Davies, Editor, *Health Service Journal*[7]

The quotations from both Joseph Kimble and Peter Davies illustrate again that plain language can encourage clearer thinking. Plain language works for any level of complexity – but only if you have thought through and understand the message you are trying to get across.

PLAIN LANGUAGE SEEN AS CONDESCENDING

Perhaps because some people think plain language is simplistic, another objection to its use is that plain language makes you sound condescending to the reader/listener. Cynics sometimes refer to communicating in plain language as 'dumbing down' (more buzz words!). There are various arguments and pieces of evidence to suggest that this concern too is unfounded (*see* Box 4.2).

Box 4.2: Evidence that plain language is not intrinsically condescending

- Box 3.4 contained just a few of the numerous examples of people preferring communications in plain language. It seems unlikely that they would prefer language that made them feel they were being patronised
- The Inland Revenue commissioned research into the views of 50 owners of small businesses on its redesigned Pay As You Earn Guidance Booklet. Among various findings, the plain language style of the booklet was liked and not considered to be condescending[8]
- In a study asking contractors and officials to comment on a revised Property Services Agency booklet, the plain language version was not considered condescending. In fact, the easier the document was to use, the better received it was[8]
- No one would accuse George Orwell, Mark Twain or any of the other eminent authors whose work is in plain English of being condescending
- Every day, millions of people buy tabloid newspapers, which tend to use plain English. People would not spend money on these if they were made to feel patronised
- Plain English is what most of us talk most of the time outside work – yet we would not generally think we were (or would be thought to be) patronising our audience

---

In short, it seems unlikely that the plain language style itself makes people feel they are being patronised. This feeling is, in fact, far more likely to result from the attitude of the writer/speaker, which is obvious in any language, whether jargon ridden or plain.

USING JARGON TO FIT IN

In linguistics (the scientific study of language), there is a technical term 'accommodation'. This describes a natural phenomenon in which people with different dialects (either geographical or social class related), when talking to each other, tend to change their own speech unconsciously to sound more like the other person's. Studies have shown changes in various areas of language, including vocabulary, grammar, pronunciation and the speed of speech. This means that if there is a core of people who use jargon, then others who are normally less inclined to do so may well start to in their presence. Although buzz words are particularly contagious, this also applies to the other types of jargon.

As well as the unconscious process of accommodation, people do sometimes intentionally modify the language they would normally use to fit in with others. A survey at ScottishPower showed that 20% of people admitted using jargon they did not understand just to fit in at work.[9]

Happily, both of these phenomena mean that if more people can be persuaded to use plain language, then this effect too will be catching. These reasons for negative jargon use therefore become less and less prevalent as more people are persuaded to use plain language.

JARGON AS A HABIT

Although people new to an environment will notice jargon, its use becomes a habit after a while. We just forget that our audience is not familiar with the language we are using. Like other habits, we do not know we are doing it until someone complains about it or asks us to explain in simpler language – which they may well not do, for fear of looking stupid.

The solution to this is to raise NHS communicators' awareness of the language they use by presenting them with evidence of their negative jargon use. Box 4.3 shows some possible sources of this, together with their relevance to an individual's or department's negative jargon use.

Generally speaking, the more directly relevant the evidence is, the better – provided it is handled sensitively, since 'directly relevant' can also be seen as 'most personal'. The problem with the less directly relevant sources is that those using jargon negatively may not believe (or want to believe) that their language use is problematic. Negative jargon use is one of those things we all love to hate, yet most of us are guilty of at least sometimes. We will not admit (even to ourselves) that we can spout jargon with the best of them.

Box 4.3: Possible sources of evidence of negative jargon use

Most directly relevant

Least directly relevant

- The results of testing the target audience's likely understanding of a particular communication
- Your own survey of what the actual target audience does or does not understand in general
- Other people's surveys of similar target audiences

Chapters 9 and 10 describe methods of testing the target audience's likely understanding of a particular communication, for written and spoken language respectively. Box 4.4 gives two examples of surveys by other people of target audiences that may be broadly similar to yours.

Box 4.4: Surveys of NHS target audiences

Example 1

In 1997, the former North West Anglia Health Authority surveyed local people who, for six months, had been involved in public meetings and discussions about the NHS, and had received briefing papers from the health authority.[10] This showed that many people did not understand, or misunderstood, common NHS jargon. For example:

- 36% of respondents believed 'primary care' meant 'life-saving services in the NHS', and a further 18% thought the term meant 'care delivered to children under 11'.
- 51% thought 'secondary care' meant 'less urgent services'
- 66% did not know what 'CPN' stood for
- 55% did not know what 'triage' meant, or believed it meant 'treating people at home not hospital'.

Yet the briefing papers these participants had received contained all these terms.

Example 2

Another piece of research, commissioned by the Central Office of Information in 1995, looked at how well recent claimants of Attendance Allowance and healthcare staff understood words and phrases used in these forms.[8] Some findings relate to terms that would be unlikely to be used in NHS communications, but others are relevant. For example, participants thought:

- 'disabled' person did not include people with a mental illness or handicap
- 'in-patient' covered anyone attending a hospital, even as an out-patient
- 'residential home' meant the home people lived in, as opposed to a communal home for older people or people with disabilities.

IMPLEMENTING PLAIN LANGUAGE SEEN AS TOO MUCH TROUBLE FOR TOO LITTLE REWARD

Finally, the idea of implementing plain language can seem unappealing because people think:

- it will be expensive to do so
- it will be time consuming to do so
- the organisation has gone, or is going, through a lot of change already
- language is a trivial concern, while there are other bigger and more important issues to deal with.

Box 4.5 shows some possible responses to these objections.

Box 4.5: Responses to the belief that implementing plain English is too much trouble for too little reward

- Although it takes time and money to implement plain language, you do not need excessive amounts of either. Your investment should in any case lead to significant savings in time and money for the organisation (*see* Box 3.2)
- During times of change, effective communications (both internal and external) are more important than ever. By improving communication, plain language can help you manage change
- Language can often seem like a relatively trivial part of management, but it is central to effective communications. Without clear communications, you may well be wasting effort invested in other management work
- Communicating is not a cheap business. For example, the National Audit Office estimates that: 'one of a kind' letters cost an organisation £20, standard letters £3.50, each page produced by senior managers from £20 to £100 or more, and each printed page on each desk £1.[11] If these communications do not get the message across effectively, then a lot of money is wasted. Research carried out by the Adult Literacy and Basic Skills Unit in 1993 showed that sloppy letter writing costs the UK £6 billion a year.[12] So language does matter

CONVINCING PEOPLE THROUGHOUT THE ORGANISATION

As with all types of change, convincing some (or even most) people that change is desirable does not lead to change if a few others who hold positions of power do not agree. To implement plain language, you need the top management team to be committed to the change. But there are probably many others in the organisation who have some role in checking the work of NHS communicators before the target audience gets to read or hear it, for example line managers and committees or other groups. Unless everyone involved in producing or agreeing communications is convinced of the value of plain language, a plain draft can rapidly become jargon ridden as it goes through the organisation.

Finally, do not forget new recruits to the organisation. Induction programmes can tell people about, and train them in, the organisation's plain language approach.

REFERENCES

1   Fowler HW (revised by Gowers E) (1983) *A Dictionary of Modern English Usage* (2e). Oxford University Press, Oxford.
2   Gowers E (revised by Greenbaum S and Whitcut J) (1986) *The Complete Plain Words* (3e). HMSO, London.
3   Kimble J (1994–95) Answering the critics of plain language. *The Scribes Journal of Legal Writing.* **5**.
4   Cutts M (1999) *Plain English Guide: how to write clearly and communicate better.* Oxford University Press, Oxford.
5   Kimble J (1996–97) Writing for dollars, writing to please. *The Scribes Journal of Legal Writing.* **6**.
6   Crystal D (1988) *The English Language*. Penguin, London.
7   Davies P (2000) Plain thinking about plain words. *Health Service Journal.* **110** (5694): 17.
8   Kempson E and Moore N (1994) *Designing Public Documents: a review of research.* Policy Studies Institute, London.
9   Plain English Campaign (2000) The business of jargon. *Plain English.* **44**: 2.
10 North West Anglia Health Authority (1998) *The Health of Wisbech: communications and information questionnaire carried out by the Public Engagement Group: report of findings.* North West Anglia Health Authority, Peterborough.
11 Wright N (2000) Cost savings from plain language (visited 30 June 2000). http://www.plainlanguage.gov/library/savings.htm
12 Plain English Campaign (1993) *The Plain English Story* (3e). Plain English Campaign, Stockport.

CHAPTER 5

INVOLVING PEOPLE IN LINKING RESEARCH TO PRACTICE

So you have convinced enough of the right people that communicating in plain language is both acceptable and beneficial. How do you now go about implementing plain language use?

Wye and McClenahan[1] found that the project teams they studied often organised large workshops or presentations and issued clinical guidelines. These approaches were successful in raising awareness of the project and of the relevant research evidence, but did not in themselves usually change behaviour. They found that putting research evidence into practice was most effective; their approach is summarised in Box 5.1.

Box 5.1: Features of an approach more likely to lead to clinical behavioural change[1]

- Using a non-threatening, face-to-face approach
- Meeting with practitioners one to one or in small groups (e.g. as a practice or clinical team)
- Relating the ideal (i.e. research evidence) to practice
- Planning for ways to improve practice
- Repeatedly going back to identify and overcome practical difficulties as they arise

All these features of an approach more likely to lead to clinical behavioural change are also relevant to bringing about change in language use.

TRAINING

Perhaps the most common way of trying to change how people communicate in organisations is one-off group training in plain language guidelines. Good trainers will tailor the training to participants' needs as far as possible, and use techniques to help people retain what they have learned. However, there are similarities between one-off group training and the large workshops or presentations described by Wye and McClenahan. Some plain language consultants say that with training alone, employees lose about 97% of what they learned within two weeks of the session.[2] This is not because of any inherent failing of the training, but simply because participants' linguistic habits and beliefs are too deeply rooted. Also, various cultural factors in the organisation may reinforce the jargon-ridden style.

If you have prepared the ground properly before starting the training phase – that is, by convincing enough of the right people that using plain language is acceptable and beneficial – then this loss should be significantly less. Using advanced courses or coaching sessions to train a few key individuals to a higher level may also help. They can then help promote the benefits of plain language, and provide follow-up support to individuals who have received the more basic training.

But most experts on implementing plain language in organisations still believe that training, although an essential part of the change process, is not enough in itself.

STYLE GUIDES

Style guides are a common way of reinforcing guidelines learned in training, and may sometimes even be used as a substitute for training. Style guides cover areas of language use where there are no right or wrong answers. These are the areas where, without such a guide, people's personal preferences and habits prevail. Typical areas include those listed in Box 5.2.

Box 5.2: Typical areas included in style guides

- The use of capital or lower-case letters, e.g. 'NHS Trust' or 'NHS trust'
- The explanation of abbreviations and acronyms. For example, most

people would agree that when you first use a term, you should write it out in full. But opinion varies as to whether you should:

— put the shortened form in brackets after it is first used, e.g. 'primary care groups (PCGs)'

— not put the shortened form in brackets after the term is first used, but just switch to it at the next mention, leaving the reader to work out that it is an abbreviation or acronym of a term mentioned in full earlier. (The *Health Service Journal*, for example, uses this style.)

- Contentious issues of grammar, such as using verbs in the plural with collective nouns (words that refer to a group of people or things, but are singular in form), e.g. 'the Health Authority is' or 'the Health Authority are'

- Equality in language, e.g. whether to use the generic 'he' (to apply to people of either sex), 'he or she', or 'they'

Style guides set down decisions on areas such as these, in the form of rules, ordered alphabetically or by theme, which together make up a 'house style'. Their main purpose is to make the communications coming from one organisation consistent.

You can also include plain language guidelines in a style guide. This is a good way of recording them in a central document that everyone can then refer to. There is an example of a style guide that includes guidelines on plain language in Part Four. You can either develop your own short style guide like this one, or you can agree to use one of the general style guides published as books, most of which include plain language guidelines. Box 5.3 lists some examples of these, and you will find others in most bookshops. There are also various style guides published on the Internet. Some of these are also listed in Box 5.3, and you will find others through a search engine. Be cautious, however, about the quality of Internet style guides, as their authors are not necessarily well informed. Make sure too that they are relevant to British English. (Many are produced by Americans, for American English.)

Box 5.3: Some examples of published style guides

- Allen RE (ed) (1990) *Oxford Writers' Dictionary*. Oxford University Press, Oxford.

- Bryson B (1997) *Troublesome Words*. Penguin, London.
  (This book is useful if you are not familiar with grammatical terms. It uses them as little as possible, and explains any it does use.)

- Fowler HW (edited by Burchfield RW) (1996) *The New Fowler's Modern English Usage* (3e). Oxford University Press, Oxford.
- Greenbaum S and Whitcut J (1998) *Longman Guide to English Usage*. Longman Dictionaries Division, London.
- Manser MH (1994) *Bloomsbury Guide to Better English*. Bloomsbury Publishing, London.
- The Economist (1998) *The Economist Style Guide*. Profile Books, London.
- Various style guides are published on the Internet, including:

  — *The Guardian* Style Guide at:
     http://www.guardianunlimited.co.uk/styleguide/
  — The European Commission translation department's style guide at:
     http://europa.eu.int/comm/translation/en/stygd/index.htm
  — *The Economist* Style Guide used to be on the Internet, but at the time of writing is not. There are plans to re-introduce it, but no definite date has been set. It would be worth keeping your eyes open for it at
     http://www.economist.com

The advantages of using a published style guide are that it is likely to be much more comprehensive and it saves the work of developing your own. The reverse side, however, is that:

- not having to go through the process of agreeing a style guide of their own may mean people are less committed to using it
- the length of the style guide may put people off referring to it and may dilute the importance you wish to place on plain language. Although there are books that focus specifically on plain language guidelines, these tend not to cover the other useful elements of style guides, such as those listed in Box 5.2.

Another possible disadvantage is that some published style guides use grammatical or other linguistic terms that not everyone is familiar with, and so may alienate or confuse some users. If you do write your own, you should remember to explain any such jargon, even if you are familiar with it yourself.

But even short style guides developed in-house have limitations. These are listed in Box 5.4, together with some hints on minimising these drawbacks.

Box 5.4: Limitations of style guides, and some possible solutions

- **Style guides tend to be designed to apply to written language only**
  But there is no reason why you should not have a style guide for spoken language
- **Style guides will not work if you just circulate them to users**
  They need to be well explained – especially so if they are being used as a substitute for (rather than supplement to) training. In either case, make sure you explain it to everyone who will be expected to use it. If you arrange group sessions but some people do not attend, for example because of pressure of work, make sure you follow them up. Also, be aware that some people may feel inhibited about asking questions or saying that they do not understand elements of the style guide in front of a group of colleagues. Give them the opportunity to resolve their queries individually if necessary
- **Style guides often get put to one side, or lost**
  You need to make them easily accessible. If most people draft written communications on computer, the best way is to store the style guide on a computer drive that everyone has access to, so that they all know exactly where to find it. Even better, get it linked in with the normal document template, so that it automatically appears when someone starts a new document. As an extra reminder, and to cover spoken communications and people who prefer to draft written communications on paper, laminate copies of the style guide and put them in each office or by every desk
- **A common objection to style guides is that they stifle individuality and personal style**
  People expressing this view often do not realise that all publishers (of books and periodicals) have style guides, as do most large organisations. Style guides are an important part of ensuring a consistent corporate image, and so looking professional, just like a logo or headed paper. (No one would argue that they ought to be able to write to people on paper of their own chosen colour and design.)

  Part of the trick of convincing people of the benefits of adopting a style guide is not to make it too prescriptive. Try to focus on the things that really matter and let people do the rest their own way. Stress that plain language guidelines, as Chapter 6 will show, are not rules. You can go against them, so long you have a good reason for doing so.

  If you are checking someone else's draft communication, only suggest changes that really do make it easier for the target audience to understand. It is tempting to make changes based on your own personal preferences, style and habits, which only irritate the recipient. Also, call any suggested changes just that – not 'corrections'

- **The status of style guides is sometimes left unclear**
  But people prefer to know whether the contents are rules or guidelines. Areas such as those listed in Box 5.2 are best suited to being rules, since there is no real need for flexibility, nor anything to be gained from giving people choice. But plain language guidelines need to be just that – guidelines not rules. As Chapter 6 will show, there are always occasions where there are good reasons for not following the guideline.

  This approach also has the bonus of making the style guide seem less prescriptive – although it is important to emphasise to users that they should always have a good reason for not following the plain language guidelines

OTHER ELEMENTS NEEDED

Experts on implementing plain English generally acknowledge that training and a style guide are necessary. They should be used at an early stage, after initial preparation of the ground. But they are not enough in themselves. You need to supplement them with other activities that meet the individual needs of the people whose behaviour you are trying to change. These activities should relate the research evidence directly to their practice.

People usually prefer to know how their own communication skills are rated. Using only group training and style guides can leave people confused about whether or not they are doing all right. Staff generally appreciate regular individual feedback on how understandable their own communications are to the target audience. As with other types of feedback, this should:

- balance the negative with the positive, so as not to demotivate the recipient
- be based on measurable indicators, so individuals and the organisation can see what progress is being made. Make sure that these indicators measure what the target audience thinks, and not your own taste and style. (Box 4.3 on p. 36 showed some possible sources of evidence of the target audience's views.)

This feedback can then be used to:

- identify individual needs for training and follow-up support
- help staff identify areas they need to concentrate on. For example, they may wish to draw up their own list of the plain English guidelines they find hard to follow, to use as a check list in their own communications.

THE IMPORTANCE OF INVOLVING EVERYONE

Finally, all managers must include themselves in any assessment of language use and training needs. They are no more likely than any other NHS employee to be able to communicate in plain language without training or support.

Staff will be rapidly put off the whole initiative if managers give the impression of thinking they have perfect communication skills themselves. Even if the managers do not really think this, it is easy to give this impression inadvertently, for example by not attending training sessions due to pressure of work.

REFERENCES

1   Wye L and McClenahan J (2000) *Getting Better with Evidence: experiences of putting evidence into practice*. King's Fund Publishing, London.
2   Words at Work International (2000) Plain language (visited 30 June 2000). http://wordsatworkint1.com/plain.htm

PART THREE

PLAIN LANGUAGE GUIDELINES

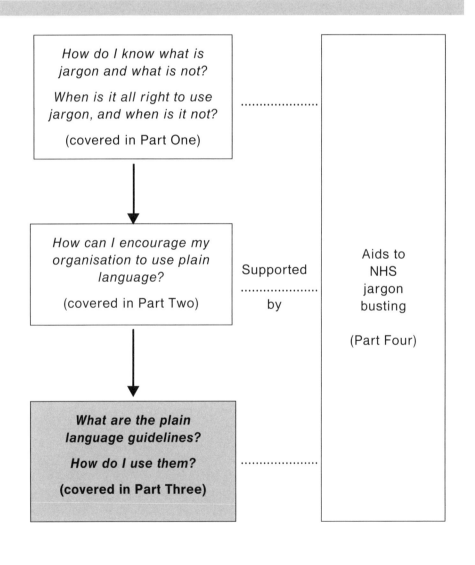

How do I know what is jargon and what is not?

When is it all right to use jargon, and when is it not?

(covered in Part One)

How can I encourage my organisation to use plain language?

(covered in Part Two)

What are the plain language guidelines?

How do I use them?

(covered in Part Three)

Supported by

Aids to NHS jargon busting

(Part Four)

CHAPTER 6

PLANNING YOUR
PLAIN DOCUMENT

The plain language movement tends to concentrate on written, paper-based communications. Although tackling jargon in speech is also important, there are fundamental differences between the processes of writing and speaking. For this reason, Chapters 6 to 9 look at plain language guidelines for writing, while Chapter 10 applies these to speech and electronic media, and to communications with audiences who have special needs.

ELEMENTS OF 'PLAIN LANGUAGE'

When we produce a document, we go through three main stages before printing and distributing it:

- planning
- writing
- testing and revising.

While the language in which we write is important, it is not the only factor that determines how well the target audience understands our message; the other stages are also vital. The term 'plain language', as used by the plain language movement, covers not only the wording of documents, but also planning, and testing and revising. The whole process is sometimes also called 'information design'.

It is the language element of plain language or information design that is most relevant to tackling jargon, and which this book concentrates on (in

Chapters 7 and 8, and Part Four). But attention to planning (covered in this chapter) will:

- help make a well-worded document even easier for the target audience to understand
- enable your organisation to realise fully the benefits described in Chapter 3.

Chapter 9 looks at testing and revising, and how to do this in a way that complements your plain language approach at the planning and writing stages.

Before turning to the plain language guidelines for each stage, a number of important basic principles are relevant to all stages.

BASIC PRINCIPLES OF THE PLAIN LANGUAGE APPROACH

GUIDELINES NOT RULES

Sometimes it seems that wherever we turn, people present us with (often ill-founded) rules for 'good' writing and 'correct' usage. But the advice contained in Chapters 6 and 7 is just that – advice (hence the term 'guidelines' as opposed to 'rules'). The guidelines suggest how to make communications more easily understandable. Just as there is evidence showing the effectiveness of plain English as a whole (as described in Chapters 3 and 4), there is also evidence for each of the guidelines that together make up the overall approach.[1]

There may be times when there are good reasons to go against the guidelines. George Orwell, suggesting five rules for good writing, concluded these with a sixth: 'Break any of these rules sooner than say anything barbarous'.[2] The important thing is that if you do go against the guidelines, you do so by design rather than by accident, and so can justify your decision. When describing guidelines, the chapters give examples of circumstances that may make it sensible to go against particular guidelines.

IMPORTANCE OF TARGET AUDIENCE

The most important principle underlying all elements of plain communication is: always think of your target audience. Some writers on plain language talk about using a 'reader-based' model. Certainly, if you always try to put yourself in the shoes of your audience when writing, you will be off to a good start.

The possible pitfall remains, however, that your familiarity with the subject matter and the jargon will cloud your judgement of the audience's needs. What is old hat to you is almost certainly brand new to some readers. Involving the target audience in developing documents is an important part of communicating in plain language. Ideally, you would involve them at all stages – planning, writing, and testing and revising. But NHS communicators producing documents are usually working to tight deadlines that just do not allow this. Although there might be certain particularly important documents where you wish to involve the audience from the beginning, for most you will do so at the testing and revising stage, if at all. Chapter 9 looks at various ways of testing documents, involving the audience to differing extents.

Another common problem NHS communicators face is having to communicate a single message to more than one type of audience: for example staff and the public or managers and clinicians. Faced with this, they often produce a document that partly meets the needs of both audiences, but fully meets the needs of neither. It can be more effective – and often no more time-consuming – to produce a number of slightly different documents, each tailored to one target audience. If you do have to produce a single document for a mixed audience, aim it at the least informed. Do not worry about boring the experts. If the document is plain, they will be able to skim through it quickly, picking out the information that is new and relevant to them.

PLAIN LANGUAGE RESOURCES

Box 6.1 lists some useful general reference books on plain English. The style guides listed in Box 5.3 also contain some basic guidance on communicating clearly, but those in Box 6.1 cover the plain English guidelines more specifically and more comprehensively.

Box 6.1: Some useful general reference books on plain English

- Hartley J (1994) *Designing Instructional Text* (3e). Kogan Page, London.
  (This book covers all elements of plain language, but is particularly strong on layout and design)
- Bailey EP (1996) *Plain English at Work: a guide to writing and speaking.* Oxford University Press, New York.

(This book is unusual in that it covers jargon in speech too – but only in prepared presentations)

- Collinson D, Kirkup G, Kyd R and Slocombe L (1992) *Plain English* (2e). Open University Press, Milton Keynes.
- Cutts M (1999) *Plain English Guide: how to write clearly and communicate better*. Oxford University Press, Oxford.
  (This classic book is particularly user-friendly and comprehensive, and is inexpensive)
- Gowers E (revised by Greenbaum S and Whitcut J) (1986) *The Complete Plain Words* (3e). HMSO, London.
- Plain English Campaign (1993) *The Plain English Story* (3e). Plain English Campaign, Stockport.
- The websites of the organisations listed in Box 2.2 include guidance on plain English. In particular, the Plain English Campaign's site includes two booklets, *How to write letters in plain English* and *How to write reports in plain English*.
- The website of the European Commission's 'Fight the FOG' campaign also includes a short course on plain English, at http://europa.eu.int/comm/translation/en/ftfog/course.htm, and a booklet on writing clearly at http://europa.eu.int/comm/translation/en/ftfog/booklet/index.htm.

PLANNING: PLAIN ENGLISH GUIDELINES

This involves:

- setting the brief (as Tim Albert calls it[3])
- structuring the information
- considering layout and design.

SETTING THE BRIEF AND STRUCTURING THE INFORMATION

Boxes 6.2 and 6.3 summarise the plain English guidelines on setting the brief and structuring your document.

Box 6.2: Plain English guidelines on setting the brief

- Decide what you want to achieve from producing the document
- Identify your target audience

- Agree a clear and honest message that the audience needs and/or wants to know. Remember that the more motivated people are to read a document, the easier they will find it. If you are not sure about the audience's needs, you can always ask them (*see* Chapter 9). If you are producing a document on behalf of a group, or that will have to be approved by a group, agreeing the message before you start is especially important. Try to make yourself leave out any unnecessary detail

- Choose the medium that is most likely to get your message across to the target audience. Examples of written media include documents, websites, emails and posters. Again, it is worth asking the audience what medium they prefer, for example whether they read newspapers regularly, and if they do, which ones

Box 6.3: Plain English guidelines on structuring your document

- As well as planning a clear message, you need to plan a clear structure for your document, grouping related ideas together and presenting information in a logical order. As you prepare your document, you need to think about what you are writing. It can help to talk to yourself (inside your head or aloud, depending on which you find more useful – and whether you share an office!). When you feel the argument is getting confusing or vague, say to yourself, 'What I really mean is...'. This can help pull from your mind the idea that was not getting through to the paper
- For the document as a whole, and for the paragraphs and sentences within it, try to present the most important information first, then support or explain it afterwards. (Note: Scientific writing traditionally works the other way round, presenting the supporting information first, and the most important information last. Doctors and other health professionals may therefore have to make a particular effort to follow this guideline)
- Think of ways to help the audience find their way around the document. Examples of such 'navigational aids' include contents pages, purpose statements, executive summaries, numbers (for pages and/or sections), headings, running headers and footers (i.e. text that appears at the top or bottom of all pages belonging to a certain section) and indexes
- Keep paragraphs and sections reasonably short. Around 100 words per paragraph is about right – so about four or five sentences. If you

> use the grammar checker in your word-processing package, the readability statistics it gives after checking may well include the average number of sentences per paragraph
> - Use examples and simple graphics (such as tables, pictures, graphs and diagrams) where these help communicate your message more clearly than words alone. Given the wide range of possible graphics, and different audiences, there are no simple rules to help you predict what your audience will find useful or confusing. This is an area where testing your graphic on members of the target audience is probably the best bet
> - Avoid including cross-references to other documents unless you are sure that your audience is familiar with these, and will have copies easily to hand

CONSIDERING LAYOUT AND DESIGN

Laying out written text in the right way helps readers to find their way through it, seeing clearly the intended structure of the document.

Some NHS documents (for example, annual reports) are professionally designed (by a graphic designer) and reproduced (by a printer). If you plan to use a graphic designer and printer for a document, they should be able to provide expert advice on the additional aspects of design that then become relevant, for example:

- format (i.e. paper and page size, and folding and stapling arrangements)
- paper weight (i.e. the thickness of the paper, measured in grams per square metre, gsm) and finish (e.g. glossy, matt or textured)
- use of colour (for text and/or background)
- leading and kerning (the space between lines and letters, both of which are set automatically by word processors)
- design of the cover.

The majority of the graphic designer's and printer's work will come after you have written and revised your text. But it makes sense to involve them at the planning stage. Their advice might affect the way you go about the writing stage, and so save time and trouble later on.

However, most NHS documents are produced in-house, using word-processing software, and then photocopied. Box 6.4 summarises the plain English guidelines that are relevant to laying out word-processed text yourself.

Whether your document is going to be reproduced professionally or in-house, you should refer to the NHS Identity Guidelines, which are available at http://www.dihnet.org.uk/nhsidentity/index.htm. These aim to give all NHS publications a consistent appearance, and also provide useful advice on projecting the right image. For example, it is important to balance the need for communications to look professional with the need for them not to look as if too much public money has been spent.

Box 6.4: Plain English guidelines on laying out and designing your document

- **Font style**
  Fonts can be 'serif' or 'sans serif'. A 'serif' is the name for the small stroke that some fonts have at the end of most letters. For example, Times New Roman is a serif font. 'Sans serif' means 'without serifs'. Arial is a sans serif font. People used to think that serif fonts were easier to read, believing that the serifs guide the reader's eye through the text. But recent research suggests there is little difference.[2] The important thing is not to use lots of different fonts within the same document. Many designers recommend using no more than two fonts – often a serif one for the body text, and a sans serif one for headings.

  Fonts can affect not only the ease of reading a text, but also the impression it gives. This is sometimes called the 'semantic property' (as opposed to the 'functional property') of a font. Serif fonts are thought to give a more classic and traditional feel to the text, while sans serif ones make it look cleaner and more modern

- **Font size**
  For a general readership, use font size 10 to 12. The best choice of font size within this range depends on the line length and number of columns you are using. Lines should be 8 to 12 words long. If you are using A4 paper, and one column (the most common format for documents produced in-house), use font size 12. If you want to use two columns (the maximum number recommended for A4 paper), use font size 10.

  Resist the temptation to reduce your font size because you cannot fit all your text on the page. Get rid of some words rather than risk making it unreadable! Use bigger font sizes for headings, with different sizes to indicate the hierarchy of headings. For example, you might use font size 16 for main headings, and size 14 for sub-headings. Make sure that you are consistent with these. This will help show the reader the structure of the text

- **White space**
  Use white space to help show the logical structure of the document, separating unrelated parts of the text, and grouping related ones. For example, leave more space above a heading than below it, so as to separate it from the text above and link it with that below. Also, use a reasonable amount of white space (for example, ample margins and space between sections) to avoid the text looking crammed on to the page.
  To get an idea of how effectively you have used white space, change the view of your word-processing screen (to about 35%) so that you can see a whole page at once. If you are looking at a paper copy of your work, do so from a distance

- **Creating emphasis**
  Where you can, create emphasis in body text through language and structure, rather than using bold or italic font, underlining or capitals. If you do need to do this, use bold or italics rather than underlining or capitals, but be sparing. Bold stands out more than italics, but both are hard to read in any quantity. Underlined text and text in capitals is particularly difficult to read, and people often think it looks unattractive

- **Justification**
  Text can be left-aligned, right-aligned or justified. This paragraph is justified, which means that all full lines of type start and finish at the same place. Many people think justified text looks neater and more professional, perhaps because most newspapers and books use it.
  In left-aligned text, all lines start at the same place, but the right-hand edge of the text is ragged. This paragraph is an example of left-aligned text. Some people say that left-aligned text is the easiest of all to read but recent research shows that it does not really matter whether you use left aligned or justified.[2]
  In right-aligned text, all lines finish at the same place, but the left-hand edge of the text is ragged. This paragraph is an example of right-aligned text. Right-aligned text is harder to read than left-aligned or justified

- **Paper weight and finish**
  For documents produced in-house, the choice of weight and finish is usually limited by the paper having to be able to pass easily through printers and/or photocopiers. Plain language experts recommend using matt paper thick enough that the print does not show from the other side

- **Use of colour**

  Producing documents in-house with coloured print is only likely to be a realistic option (in terms of time and money) if you have a colour printer (and perhaps colour photocopier) and do not need many copies. Another way of introducing colour more easily is to use coloured paper, with black print.

  If using colour in either of these ways, do so for a reason rather than just for the sake of it, and make sure there is a strong contrast between the colour of the type and the background

Just as a style guide is a useful way to reinforce the language element of plain English, so you can help staff to follow the guidelines on layout by creating a template (or adjusting the normal template) in the organisation's word-processing software. This will then automatically do many of the things listed in Box 6.4. You could create different templates for documents for different purposes and audiences, and of different types and lengths. Templates work best where people draft their documents directly on to a word processor (which seems to be increasingly common). But even those who draft manually or on audiotape eventually need their work typed up, and the template can be used at that stage. Make sure you set up some training on where to find the template and how to use it. Also, make someone available to provide individual support to template users following initial training.

REFERENCES

1   Kempson E and Moore N (1994) *Designing Public Documents: a review of research*. Policy Studies Institute, London.
2   Crystal D (1987) *The Cambridge Encyclopedia of Language*. Cambridge University Press, Cambridge.
3   Albert T (1992) *Medical Journalism: the writer's guide*. Radcliffe Medical Press, Oxford.

CHAPTER 7

WRITING PLAINLY

Be short, be simple, be human.[1] This was Sir Ernest Gowers' advice on communicating plainly in his classic book *The Complete Plain Words*. These same principles underpin all the guidelines on writing plainly, which this chapter explains.

Writing in plain English may seem like hard work to start with, but do not despair. Like everything else, it becomes easier with practice. And just as jargon is catching, so is plain English – both within your own writing, and from yours to other people's.

- If you start a document in plain language, it becomes increasingly natural to carry on in the same style.
- If you communicate in plain language, then others will increasingly do so too.

DOES GRAMMAR MATTER?

Some people think that plain language is about promoting perfect grammar; others think that it is about letting grammar slip. Neither view is right. Plain language is in fact about taking a common-sense approach to grammar – being correct, without being pedantic about 'rules' that really do not matter (like infinitive splitting, discussed in Chapter 4).

Real grammar is vital to clear communication. It is a basic set of rules which, by prescribing how words and sentences are put together, enables us to understand each other. Poor grammar may well impair understanding because it leads to ambiguous or confusing language. It is also distracting for readers who know the rules, and often stops them from concentrating on the message itself.

The extent to which you are aware of, and comfortable with, grammar rules is largely a matter of luck. It is partly natural aptitude, but whether or not you were taught grammar formally at school makes a big difference too. You can partly remedy a lack of knowledge of grammar rules through training (for example, by one of the organisations listed in Box 2.2). Reading and referring to a good basic grammar book (*see* Box 7.1) can also help. Common errors can be included in the organisation's style guide (as they are in the example of a short style guide in Part Four).

Grammar checkers in word-processing packages can also be useful, but need to be treated with caution. For all their clever features, computers are still poor at understanding language. If you are not already reasonably familiar with grammar, you will not know when the checker is giving wrong advice (as they often do). If you are not confident in your own grammar ability, you may not have the nerve to ignore its advice. Often an approachable colleague who is good at grammar is a far better bet for having a quick check through your document.

Another possibility – ideally as an addition rather than a substitute for a human's advice – is to buy more sophisticated grammar-checking software. Stylewriter–the Plain English Editor has a good reputation. It is quick and easy to use, and picks up many style and usage problems missed by other grammar checkers. It has the added advantage of being geared to a plain English style. You can find out more about this software from the Plain Language Commission (*see* Box 2.2).

In summary, although it is probably a good idea to make some effort to get reasonably up to scratch on basic grammar, you probably have far more pressing things to do. You could put in a lot of time and not move forward much. So go on a one-day course, get a good book and possibly a better grammar checker, make the most of your colleagues' skills – and then stop worrying about it.

Box 7.1: Useful books on basic grammar

- Alexander LG (1993) *The Essential English Grammar*. Addison Wesley Longman ELT Division, London.
- Crystal D and Barton G (1996) *Discover Grammar*. Longman Schools Division, Harlow.
- Field M (2000) *Polish Up Your Punctuation and Grammar: master the basics of the English language and write with greater confidence*. How To Books, Oxford.
- Phythian BA (1992) *Teach Yourself English Grammar*, revised edn. Hodder and Stoughton Educational Division, London.

I would recommend the same approach to getting punctuation and spelling right. Do your best to be correct, to avoid confusing or distracting your audience.

Box 7.2 lists several useful guides to good punctuation.

Box 7.2: Useful guides to punctuation

- Cutts M (1999) *Plain English Guide: how to write clearly and communicate better*. Oxford University Press, Oxford.
  (This gives a simple and useful overview of good punctuation.)

The following are more detailed guides to good punctuation:

- Trask RL (1997) *The Penguin Guide to Punctuation*. Penguin, London.
- Carey GV (1976) *Mind the Stop: a brief guide to punctuation*. Penguin, London.

Misspellings are particularly hard to spot if you do not have a naturally good eye for what looks right or wrong. Even if you have, it can be hard to look objectively at your own writing. Spell checkers are more reliable than grammar checkers, but they do let through properly spelt words whose meaning may be far from what you meant. (This is when you get embarrassing mistakes like 'pubic health' for 'public health'.) Again, it is best to get someone else with a good eye for detail to do a final check.

DOES 'POLITICAL CORRECTNESS' MATTER?

Some people think that plain language is about being 'politically correct'. In fact, most books on plain English do not mention equality in language at all. And I have seen plenty of plain language rewordings, produced by recognised experts, that contain prime examples of sexism and other prejudice.

However, I believe that paying attention to equality in language is an essential part of plain language. Plain language is all about getting your message across to the target audience effectively. You may think that bothering about equality in language is trivial and unnecessary. In fact, there is plenty of research to show that language has a powerful influence on attitudes, behaviours and perceptions.[2] But it makes little business sense to offend your readers. If they are annoyed by some apparent prejudice in your document, they will be distracted from what you are trying to say.

Getting it right in this area is not always straightforward, but there are again a number of specialist books that can help (*see* Box 7.3).

Box 7.3: Useful reference books on equality in writing

- Doyle M (1995) *A-Z of Non-Sexist Language*. The Women's Press, London.
- Maggio R (1997) *Talking About People: a guide to fair and accurate language*. The Oryx Press, Phoenix, AZ.
  (This book is particularly comprehensive, as it covers all areas of prejudice, not just sexism. It also includes research evidence showing the importance of avoiding prejudice in language.)
- Miller C and Swift K (1995) *Handbook of Non-Sexist Writing for Writers, Editors and Speakers*, revised edn. The Women's Press, London.

WRITING: PLAIN ENGLISH GUIDELINES

Many people think that writing in plain English is all a matter of vocabulary, getting rid of archaic and complex words. But the length, structure and tone of sentences are just as important. The guidelines cover all these areas, as the summary in Box 7.4 shows.

Box 7.4: Writing: summary of plain language guidelines

Using plain words and phrases
1 Get rid of useless words and phrases.
2 Use short, familiar words and phrases.
3 Feel free to repeat the same word.
Using plain sentences
4 Aim for an average sentence length of 15 to 20 words.
5 Use verbs rather than abstract nouns where possible.
6 Prefer active to passive verbs.
7 Write in the first and second person where you can.
8 Use positive rather than negative statements.

To write plainly, you need to apply all the guidelines to your language. However, to illustrate each guideline simply and clearly for this section, the examples in each show how they would change if you applied that guideline only. Chapter 8 looks at combining all the guidelines to tackle NHS jargon effectively, and completes the process of making plain the examples used here.

You can see further examples of applying each guideline in the example of a short style guide in Part Four.

Using plain words and phrases

Guideline 1: Get rid of useless words and phrases

You can often get rid of some words altogether, without affecting the meaning of your message. This instantly shortens your document.

When preparing a document, try to look critically at it, removing words and seeing whether the meaning is really affected. For example, the following sentences can easily lose several words (as shown by the lines through these).

> ~~In total~~ *20 individuals were identified across three trusts,* ~~with the number~~
> ~~of key people identified~~ *ranging from five to eight in each* ~~trust~~.
> (from a research and development project report)
> ~~The nature of the problem is such that~~ *the likelihood of system and*
> *equipment failures is often difficult to predict.*
> (from a trust's summary business plan)

Box 7.5 shows some examples of words and phrases that you can often get rid of without changing your message.

Box 7.5: Words and phrases that are often useless

- in total
- a total of
- absolutely
- very
- quite
- actually
- basically
- at the end of the day

- to all intents and purposes
- current
- currently
- existing
- in due course
- in other words
- obviously
- of course

Guideline 2: Use short, familiar words and phrases

Generally speaking, shorter words are more familiar than longer ones. Of the 200 most frequently used words in English, 174 have just one syllable, with 24 two-syllable words and just two three-syllable ones.[3]

As with all guidelines, there are exceptions.

- Some longer words may be familiar to most people (for example 'immediately', 'encourage', 'honesty', 'suspicious', 'practical', 'benefit'). Longer words like these are fine to use, so long as you are sure they really will be familiar to all members of your target audience. But if there is a shorter word, you may as well use this, as it is likely to be even easier to understand.

- Other longer words may be less familiar, but are the only ones that can explain exactly what you mean. For words like these, you should take the same approach as you would for technical jargon (which is also not easily replaceable) – use it, but if the audience will not understand it, explain the meaning in plain language (*see* Chapter 8). Do not expect the audience to look words up in the dictionary. Even if they have access to one, they will almost certainly not bother to do so, and your message will be lost.
- Some words may be short but unfamiliar. This includes many foreign words, particularly Latin ones, which you should avoid using. Some (for example 'vice versa', 'per cent', 'etc.') have become so common that most people understand them. But others (such as 'per se', 'sic' and 'ceteris paribus') are not easily understood. Also, as mentioned in Chapter 1, buzz words are often short but obscure.

Knowing what is familiar to your target audience is not always straightforward. The following tips may help.

- Short, familiar words tend to be of Anglo-Saxon (Old English) rather than Romance (Latin) origin. Of the 1000 most frequently used English words, 83% are Anglo-Saxon.[3] This may not mean much to those who have not studied languages. But if you have done some German (or perhaps Dutch or Scandinavian), English words that are similar to words from these languages are often of Anglo-Saxon origin. Similarly, if you know French, Spanish or Italian, English words that are similar to words from these languages are often of Romance origin.
- An easier way of knowing what words to use is to think of what words you would use in everyday conversation.
- It can also be useful to use a thesaurus (either in paper or electronic form – there is one in Microsoft Word) to remind yourself of short alternatives to longer words. The lists of examples of NHS buzz words and gobbledegook in Part Four should also help.
- If in doubt about what is familiar to your audience, ask some of them. (Chapter 9 looks at this in more detail.)

The following examples show how replacing long, unusual words with shorter, more familiar ones helps to make language clearer.

Before: 'Scientific studies have convinced most people nowadays that smoking is deleterious not only to them but also to others who share their company.'
(from a health authority's public health annual report)

After: 'Scientific studies have convinced most people nowadays that smoking is bad not only for them but also for others who share their company.'

Before: 'The day's proceedings will be documented in order to inform operational planning and policy making.'
(from details of a conference for NHS managers and service users)
After: 'The day's events will be noted down in order to inform operational planning and policy making.'

Sometimes two or more words (not always long, unfamiliar ones themselves) combine to make a long or unfamiliar phrase. Treat these phrases in the same way: replace them with shorter, more familiar alternatives. For example, in the following sentence, 'the rationale behind its procurement' could be replaced by the more readily understandable 'why it had bought it'.

'The Trust took the decision to demonstrate the equipment to as many of its staff as possible, to inform them of its capabilities and the rationale behind its procurement.'
(from a trust's annual report)

Guideline 3: Feel free to repeat the same word

One of the 'rules' that many of us were taught by our English teachers was that it was 'bad English' to use the same word twice within some randomly defined area – be it a sentence, several lines, or the same paragraph. (This 'rule' is sometimes known as 'elegant variation'.) It is true that repetition can lead to an unnecessarily wordy style. But it is always better to repeat a word than to use synonyms that are not plain, or that may make the reader wonder whether you are talking about the same thing or something different.

For example, in the following paragraph, 'older people' is unnecessarily replaced by the longer-winded 'elderly individuals'. Using 'older people' again would be perfectly acceptable, and much plainer.

'The health of older people often deteriorates gradually, giving some opportunity for crisis prevention. There is said to be a need for a simple method of targeting the subgroup of elderly individuals who are at particular risk and on whom preventive programmes should focus.'
(from a health authority's annual report)

In the following passage, the Day Care Unit is said to be 'operational', when just plain 'open' would do. It really does not matter that the word 'opening' has been used in the previous sentence.

'This time last year, we were busy making preparations for the opening of the Day Care Unit. It has now been operational since last Easter, taking more patients and with more facilities in a "made-to-measure" environment.'
(from a hospice's newsletter)

USING PLAIN SENTENCES

Guideline 4: Aim for an average sentence length of 15 to 20 words

The longer a sentence, the more concentration is needed, putting a greater burden on the reader's short-term memory. Also, long sentences often contain more complex structures.[4]

Sentences should be an average of 15 to 20 words, with some longer and some shorter sentences for variety and effect. For example, shorter sentences are useful for emphasis. In each sentence, make one or perhaps two points. If you use the grammar checker in your word-processing package, the readability statistics it gives after checking will probably include the average number of words per sentence.

If editing existing text, there are two easy ways of dealing with sentences that are too long.

- Divide them into a larger number of shorter sentences. This is a good solution when you can see that the long sentence is made up of two or more separate statements (often joined by 'and' or 'but').
  Example (using the first example of gobbledegook from Chapter 1)
  Before: 'It was noted that cash from the management underspend has been identified to support the plan but there was concern that if there were no monies available in the future, interest would drop and the plan would not be delivered.'
  After: 'It was noted that cash from the management underspend has been identified to support the plan. But there was concern that if there were no monies available in the future, interest would drop and the plan would not be delivered.'
  (Note: Many people are taught at school not to start a sentence with 'and' or 'but'. But, as Chapter 4 noted, it is in fact fine to do so, as you will see from published style guides such as those listed in Box 5.3. This style is particularly common in journalistic writing – have a look in the broadsheet national newspapers.)
- If the sentence contains a list of items, rearrange these as bullet points.
  Example (using the second example of gobbledegook from Chapter 1)
  Before: 'Directors are asked to note the current position, be aware that there are likely to be further developments in the situation in coming

months and endorse the action taken so far to address our paramount concern, which is the health and well being of local residents.'
After: 'Directors are asked to:

- note the current position
- be aware that there are likely to be further developments in the situation in coming months
- endorse the action taken so far to address our paramount concern, which is the health and well being of local residents.'

Guideline 5: Use verbs rather than abstract nouns where possible

Many nouns (words that refer to people, places or things) are formed from verbs (words that express actions, states and events), for example 'preparation' (from the verb 'to prepare'), 'decision' (from 'to decide') and 'application' (from 'to apply'). The technical term for this sort of noun, derived from a verb, is a 'deverbal noun'. Deverbal nouns are usually abstract rather than concrete (that is, they refer to intangible things, rather than material objects). They quite often end in '-ion'.

One of the reasons that gobbledegook sounds dull is that it uses deverbal nouns instead of their equivalent verbs. These also make the text more difficult to read.

Try to use verbs where you can. Because verbs express actions, they make text sound more vigorous. The following sentences illustrate this. The nouns underlined can all be easily turned into verbs, giving a more lively style.

Before: 'Jane was gladdened by the <u>improvement</u> the children had shown even after such a relatively short space of time.'
(from a trust's patient newsletter)
After: 'Jane was gladdened by how much the children had improved even after such a relatively short space of time.'

Before: 'The Trust is undertaking a thorough <u>review</u> of its activities to ensure <u>compliance</u> with existing and forthcoming <u>provision</u> in the Disability Discrimination Act.'
(from a trust board paper)
After: 'The Trust is thoroughly reviewing its activities to ensure it complies with what the Disability Discrimination Act provides for, now and in the future.'
(Note: you will often find that when you change a word or phrase in an existing sentence, you have to change other words, or even parts of its structure, for it still to make sense. For example, when you change 'provision' to 'provides for' in the sentence above, you cannot keep the

phrase 'existing and forthcoming'. You have to change this to something like 'now and in the future'.)

Guideline 6: Prefer active to passive verbs

When a verb is active, the sentence always includes the person or thing doing the action (which we can call the 'doer'). This is followed by the verb, and then the person or thing that is on the receiving end of the action (the 'recipient'). For example, the following sentence is active:

doer	verb	recipient
The Trust	*produced*	*a document.*

When a verb is passive, the recipient comes first, followed by the verb. The doer may or may not then be included.

You can also spot a passive by the form of words used. A passive verb always includes part of the verb 'to be' ('am', 'are', 'is', 'be', 'being', 'was', 'were' or 'been'), followed by a 'past participle', which you can usually spot by its '-ed' or '-en' ending. If the doer is included, it is introduced by the word 'by'. For example, the passive version of the sentence analysed above would be:

recipient	verb	doer
A document	*was produced*	*by the Trust.*

But you could also miss off the doer:

recipient	verb
A document	*was produced.*

Active verbs are more consistent with plain language because:

- they use fewer words, so leading to shorter sentences
- by always including the doer, they make the document more personal and human
- stating the doer (and so being explicit about who is responsible for the action) is consistent with the plain language values of openness and honesty
- the word order places less strain on the reader's short-term memory.

Although it therefore makes sense to use active verbs wherever possible, there are situations when using the passive is sensible, such as:

- when the doer is irrelevant, unimportant, obvious or unknown, for example:
  'The main part of the hospital was built in 1977.'
  Assuming your aim was to let people know the age of the hospital (rather than who built it), it would sound odd to say instead:
  'J Bloggs & Co. built the main part of the hospital in 1977.'
     Sometimes you can avoid using a passive verb by making the doer general. For example, in a sentence starting 'It could be argued that...', you could say instead, 'Some argue that...'
- when starting the sentence with the recipient makes your message clearer and punchier. For example, you may want to focus attention on the recipient, as in the following sentence:
  'Abuse, aggression and violence towards staff will not be tolerated.'
  This sentence would lose its impact if you rephrased it, moving 'abuse, aggression and violence' to a later – and less noticeable – position:
  'We will not tolerate abuse, aggression and violence towards staff.'

In summary, try to use active verbs. Ask yourself who or what is performing the action (there may already be a 'by'-phrase in the sentence telling you), and start the sentence with this person or thing. For example, it is easy to make the following sentences active:

Before: 'A mind-mapping exercise will be undertaken by the whole group on trends around clinical governance, to share current reality and provide data for dialogue.'
(from an advertisement for a conference)
After: 'The whole group will undertake a mind-mapping exercise on trends around clinical governance, to share current reality and provide data for dialogue.'

Before: 'As we enter the third millennium, the challenge that is faced by us all is to demonstrate that the co-ordinated efforts of local organisations and local people can bring greater improvements in health and well being than if we work alone.'
(from a health improvement programme)
After: 'As we enter the third millennium the challenge that we all face is to demonstrate that the co-ordinated efforts of local organisations and local people can bring greater improvements in health and well being than if we work alone.'

If an active verb does not sound right, make sure this is because it makes your message less clear and not because of any linguistic prejudices, such as those discussed in Chapter 4. It may be particularly difficult to use active verbs in documents relating to complaints and litigation if you are to avoid admitting blame before it is proven. Although it would clearly be foolish to go against legal advice for the sake of plain language, try to follow the guideline where you sensibly can.

Guideline 7: Write in the first and second person where you can

When writing in the first person, you use the words 'I', 'me', 'we' and 'us' to refer to yourself, or your team, department or organisation. This makes the document sound more human, and engages the attention of the reader more easily. Addressing the audience for your writing in the second person (i.e. using 'you') will also help the document to sound more directly relevant, and so hold the reader's interest, as the following example shows.

> **Before:** 'The Trust recognises the importance of keeping our patients and purchasers fully informed of developments within the organisation and within the NHS nationally.'
> (from a trust's newsletter for patients and purchasers)
> **After:** 'We recognise the importance of keeping you fully informed of developments within our organisation and within the NHS nationally.'

One common objection in the NHS to using the first person is that it may not be obvious exactly who the doer is, and so who is responsible for a view, decision or action. For example, I came across a health authority whose staff were unhappy about using the first person in board papers and minutes. You can usually get around this by stating clearly at the first mention of 'I' or 'we' who exactly you mean, for example 'as director of public health, I...', 'we in the finance department...' or 'we on the Board...'

Guideline 8: Use positive rather than negative statements

Putting your points negatively makes them harder for the audience to understand. It can take some time to work out the meaning of statements that contain negative terms (such as 'not', 'none' and 'no'), particularly where more than one negative is used.

Try to phrase your points positively where you can. For example, the following sentences are clearer when rephrased positively:

> **Before:** 'The strategy will not lead to a diminution of existing core service provision.'
> (from a community safety strategy)
> **After:** 'The strategy will safeguard existing core service provision.'

Before: 'These quality improvements have not been gained lightly, but by the dedication, commitment, hard work and teamwork of all staff. Not satisfied to rest on its laurels, however, the Trust is now looking towards the European Foundation of Quality Management model as a target for the future.'
(from a trust's quality report)
After: 'These quality improvements have been gained through hard work, by the dedication, commitment and teamwork of all staff. Keen to improve further, however, the Trust is now looking towards the European Foundation of Quality Management model as a target for the future.'

There may, however, be some situations where using the negative does convey your meaning better. One example of this is in commands not to do something, such as:

'Never, ever talk about what you did in your old organisation.'

This sentence would lose much of its impact if rephrased positively:

'Always keep quiet about what you did in your old organisation.'

REFERENCES

1   Gowers E (revised by Greenbaum S and Whitcut J) (1986) *The Complete Plain Words* (3e). HMSO, London.
2   Maggio R (1997) *Talking About People: a guide to fair and accurate language*. The Oryx Press, Phoenix, AZ.
3   Gramley S and Pätzold K-M (1992) *A Survey of Modern English*. Taylor & Francis, London.
4   Hartley J (1994) *Designing Instructional Text* (3e). Kogan Page, London.

CHAPTER 8

TACKLING NHS JARGON

Few communications contain just one type of jargon. Written language often contains both technical jargon and gobbledegook, and occasionally some buzz words. This chapter shows you how to bring together the individual guidelines on writing plainly to:

- get rid of buzz words and gobbledegook, in communications for all audiences
- explain terms of technical jargon, in communications for audiences who are not familiar with these.

WRITING OR TRANSLATING?

When you first start trying to write in plain English, you may find yourself adding an extra stage. Instead of writing in plain English, you may produce a jargon-ridden draft (either in your head, or on paper or screen) and then 'translate' it. This is illustrated in Figure 8.1. (This is, in effect, an editing process, rather like the commercial service offered by plain language consultants.) This translating stage makes writing a document more time-consuming. Try to cut it out as soon as possible, drafting all text in plain English from the start.

You may also find yourself translating existing, jargon-ridden text which has been written by someone who is not familiar with the plain language guidelines. Introducing plain language to all members of your organisation, as Chapter 2 advocates, will minimise this problem.

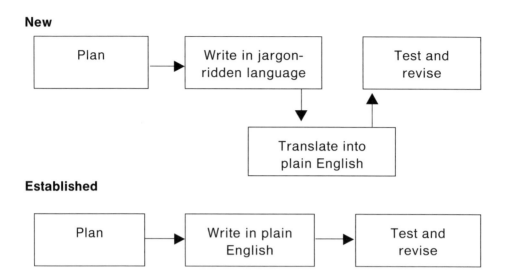

Figure 8.1   Writing processes when plain English is new, and established.

If you are translating into (as opposed to writing from scratch in) plain English, it makes sense to tackle the three different types of jargon in this order:

- buzz words
- gobbledegook
- technical jargon.

Because you need to try to get rid of buzz words and gobbledegook altogether, it makes sense to tackle these before technical jargon. And because buzz words are easier to tackle than gobbledegook (since they involve individual words and phrases only, rather than structural features too), it makes sense to tackle these first of all.

TACKLING BUZZ WORDS

Most buzz words can easily be replaced by plain words and phrases whose meaning is much clearer to most people, including other NHS communicators.

Apply the guidelines on using plain words and phrases (*see* Chapter 7) to replace buzz words with plain English alternatives. The list of examples of NHS buzz words in Part Four should help you do this.

TACKLING GOBBLEDEGOOK

Gobbledegook is more difficult to get rid of than buzz words, because it involves sentences, as well as words and phrases.

Apply the guidelines on using both plain words and phrases, and plain sentences, to communicate plainly. The list of examples of NHS gobbledegook in Part Four should help you to simplify words and phrases.

When translating someone else's text, you may come across a particularly jargon-ridden phrase, sentence or paragraph, and at first not understand the message. Even when translating your own text, you may find the process of trying to make it plain leaves you wondering exactly what message you wanted to communicate. If you find yourself getting lost in jargon like this, look away from the computer screen or paper, and say to yourself, 'What I (or the writer) really mean(s) is...' (*see* Box 6.3). As discussed in Chapter 3, being forced to think clearly about what exactly you arc trying to say can only be a good thing. It encourages clearer planning and policy making, as well as clearer communications.

TACKLING TECHNICAL JARGON

DECIDING WHAT TO EXPLAIN

The first stage in tackling technical jargon is to identify the target audience for your communication. You may be communicating with colleagues, all of whom you can reasonably expect to understand the technical jargon you plan to use. If so, then go ahead and use it freely. Be sure, however, that you are not conning yourself into believing buzz words or gobbledegook to be technical jargon.

If your audience will probably not understand NHS technical jargon, then you must think about explaining it. You do not necessarily need to explain every piece of technical jargon. You need to judge whether or not the audience will be able to understand the term well enough (for both their own and your good) without explanation. For example, the general public may be aware of the meaning of some terms through media coverage. The meaning of other terms may be obvious from the context. Be cautious with those terms that are made up of ordinary words but have taken on a different, specialist meaning (for example 'competence', 'executive letter' and 'Green Paper'). The meaning may be obvious to you and your colleagues, but could lead to serious misunderstanding by the target audience (as shown in Box 4.4). Misunderstanding terms is potentially more dangerous than not understanding them at all. People will not ask you to clarify what you mean, because they will think they know. But they may be going away with completely the wrong idea.

Do not rely on people to look up terms elsewhere (for example in a separate guide to NHS jargon) or to ask you to explain what you mean. Many people will either not bother or be too embarrassed to do this.

Judging what you do need to explain is not easy, but becomes easier with experience. Check with someone from the target audience, if you can. The list of examples of NHS technical jargon in Part Four may also help; this includes a number of common terms that need explaining.

EXPLAINING TERMS OF TECHNICAL JARGON

Once you have decided which items of technical jargon to explain, you need to think about how you will do this. There are two main possibilities, each with its pros and cons:

- explaining the term as you mention it in the communication. The advantage of this is that the audience gets an immediate explanation of what you mean, without having to look away from the document. However, if the explanation is long, it can lead to long and unwieldy sentences, or interrupt the structure of the communication. This can make your message harder to understand
- explaining the term elsewhere, for example in a footnote or glossary. The advantage of this is that you can give a more detailed explanation. The disadvantage is that the reader has to look away from the text, and so again is distracted from your message.

It is possible to combine the best parts of each of these approaches, and to avoid the disadvantages, by:

- always explaining the term as you mention it in the document, simply and concisely (in just enough detail for the reader to be able to understand your message). This may make your sentence a little longer, and although you should be careful that it does not get too long, the odd longer sentence is fine. Remember that it is the *average* sentence length that should be 15 to 20 words, not each individual sentence. Also, plain English experts advise that including a lot of information in brackets or dashes, especially in the middle of sentences, can hinder communication. This makes the structure more complex, and takes the reader's attention off the main message. You should therefore keep the explanation as brief as possible. If you need to use more than a few words to explain a piece of technical jargon, do so in a separate sentence

- providing a glossary for the audience to refer to at their leisure – only if you think it would be useful to give a more detailed explanation. This may be useful to you, in getting your message across, or to the audience, in increasing their knowledge (and so empowering them). Since you would have explained all terms briefly in the text as you mentioned them (as described above), readers would not have to refer to the glossary as they were going along to understand your message.

All explanations – both in the text and in the glossary – need to be written in plain English, following the guidelines given in Chapter 7. If you are writing both a shorter and longer explanation for a technical term, it is usually easier to do the longer one first. You will often find that you can then extract a few words straight from this, to use as the shorter one.

KNOWING WHEN TO RE-EXPLAIN TERMS

Should you re-explain a term every time it is mentioned? This depends on how the audience will use the document.

- Do you expect the document to be read from beginning to end, in order (as you may, for example, with a letter)? In this case, it is usually enough to explain terms of technical jargon the first time they appear. But you may wish to re-explain terms if there is a big gap between them. This will save readers looking back to your first explanation, if they cannot remember it.
- Will people read just one chapter or section of a document (for example, the one relevant to their own area in a document setting out health plans for different localities)? You need to explain terms the first time they appear in each section.
- Might readers dip into the document at any point, reading only small amounts of any section, not necessarily from the beginning (for example, an annual report, which a patient may pick up in a waiting room)? You should explain terms the first time they appear in each paragraph.

In other words, look at how the document as a whole divides naturally into chunks that you can count on people reading in their entirety. Explain terms of technical jargon the first time they are mentioned in each chunk.

DEALING WITH ACRONYMS AND ABBREVIATIONS

Exactly the same guidance applies to the writing out in full of acronyms and abbreviations: do so the first time people are likely to come across them. Put the short form in brackets immediately afterwards. You can set most word-processing packages to expand acronyms or abbreviations automatically. This can be useful if you are often going to have to write a short form out in full.

Just as the meaning of some technical jargon may be obvious enough to the audience without explanation, some acronyms and abbreviations, once written out in full, may not need explaining. For example, North West Anglia Health Authority found that 66% of the local people they surveyed did not know what 'CPN' stood for (*see* Box 4.4).[1] However, writing out 'CPN' as 'community psychiatric nurse (CPN)' at the first mention in a document may be enough to ensure the audience understands your message.

AGREEING EXPLANATIONS

It is not always easy to explain terms of technical jargon simply and clearly. It may be particularly difficult to get a group of people to agree on explanations. Sometimes their objections may be more to do with an aversion to, or lack of understanding of, plain English, for one of the reasons discussed in Chapter 4. In this case, you may need to convince them of the benefits of plain English. It is often especially hard to agree explanations for areas where there is a highly specialised knowledge base, for example public health and finance. Experts in such fields may find it hard to leave out the finer points of technical detail. Bear in mind too that they may also have been taught to value gobbledegook as a style of writing.

Once you have agreed explanations, it is worth recording them for future use. It may be useful to keep these as a comprehensive glossary available to all members of the organisation, perhaps in electronic form on a computer drive that everyone has access to. People writing documents can then select the explanations they need, without rewriting them each time, saving time and improving consistency between documents. Sharing the glossary with other local NHS organisations saves even more time, and ensures consistency across the whole local health system (as well as supporting partnership working).

This approach to tackling buzz words, gobbledegook and technical jargon is summarised in Figure 8.2. The diagram shows where in the book you can find the information you need to carry out each stage of tackling NHS jargon.

EXAMPLES

I applied the advice contained in this chapter to the sentences partly rewritten in Chapter 7. The results were as follows. You may think of

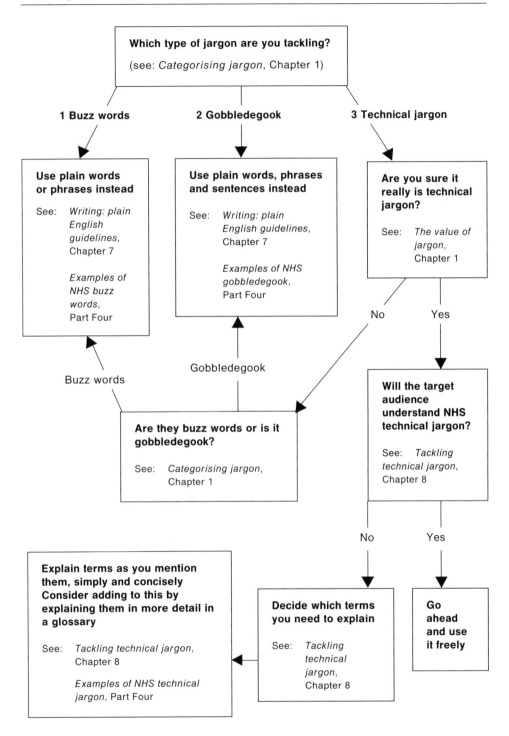

Figure 8.2 Tackling NHS jargon: summary.

clearer or more accurate alternatives. But I hope that my versions will be useful as examples of how to make sentences plainer.

EXAMPLE 1

Original sentence: 'In total 20 individuals were identified across three trusts, with the number of key people identified ranging from five to eight in each trust.'
Plain sentence: 'We picked out 20 people across three trusts (NHS organisations providing local healthcare), ranging from five to eight in each.'
What I did: In Chapter 7, I deleted the useless words 'in total', 'with the number of key people identified' and 'trust'. I have then:

- changed the long words 'individuals' and 'identified' to the shorter ones 'people' and 'picked out'
- used an active rather than a passive verb ('We picked out 20 people' instead of '20 people were picked out')
- used the first person ('We' rather than, say, 'The project team')
- added in a brief explanation of the technical jargon 'trusts'. (For this term, just as for technical terms in the other examples in this section, you might choose also to give a more detailed explanation in a glossary. You could take this from the plain English explanations of examples of NHS technical jargon, in Part Four.)

EXAMPLE 2

Original sentence: 'The nature of the problem is such that the likelihood of system and equipment failures is often difficult to predict.'
Plain sentence: 'It is often hard to predict whether systems and equipment will fail.'
What I did: In Chapter 7, I deleted the useless words 'The nature of the problem is such that'. I have then:

- changed the longer word 'difficult' to the shorter one 'hard'
- used the phrase 'whether...will fail' instead of 'the likelihood of failures', so getting rid of 'failures', a deverbal noun (noun formed from a verb – *see* Chapter 7).

EXAMPLE 3

Original sentence: 'Scientific studies have convinced most people nowadays that smoking is deleterious not only to them but also to others who share their company.'

Plain sentence: 'Scientific studies have convinced most people nowadays that smoking is bad not only for them but also for others around them.'
What I did: In Chapter 7, I changed the long and unusual word 'deleterious' to the short and familiar word 'bad'. I have then:

- simplified 'who share their company' to 'around them'.

EXAMPLE 4

Original sentence: 'The day's proceedings will be documented in order to inform operational planning and policy making.'
Plain sentence: 'We will note down the day's events to help people plan operations (the day-to-day running of the NHS) and make policy (longer-term plans).'
What I did: In Chapter 7, I changed the long words 'proceedings' and 'documented' to the shorter alternatives 'events' and 'noted down'. I have then:

- deleted the useless words 'in order'
- changed the deverbal nouns 'planning' and 'making' to the verbs 'plan' and 'make'
- changed the passive 'The day's events will be noted down' to the active 'We will note down'
- used the first person 'We'
- added in a brief explanation of the technical jargon 'operations' and 'policy'. (This is particularly important for the term 'operations', as readers could confuse its meaning here with the more common meaning of 'surgical procedures'.)

EXAMPLE 5

Original sentence: 'The Trust took the decision to demonstrate the equipment to as many of its staff as possible, to inform them of its capabilities and the rationale behind its procurement.'
Plain sentence: 'We decided to demonstrate the equipment to as many of our staff as possible. We showed them what it could do and why we had bought it.'
What I did: In Chapter 7, I simplified the phrase 'the rationale behind its procurement' to 'why it had bought it'. I have then:

- simplified the phrase 'inform them of its capabilities' to 'showed them what it could do'

- split the sentence into two, to keep the sentence length down
- changed the deverbal noun 'decision' to the verb 'decided'
- put the sentences into the first person, for example using 'We' and 'our' instead of 'The Trust' and 'its'.

EXAMPLE 6

Original sentence: 'The health of older people often deteriorates gradually, giving some opportunity for crisis prevention. There is said to be a need for a simple method of targeting the subgroup of elderly individuals who are at particular risk and on whom preventive programmes should focus.'

Plain sentence: 'The health of older people often gets worse gradually, giving us some chance to prevent crises. We need a simple method of targeting older people who are at particular risk. We can then focus preventive programmes (schemes to prevent ill health) on this group.'

What I did: In Chapter 7, I changed the words 'elderly individuals' to the plainer 'older people', despite this having been used in the previous sentence. I have then:

- got rid of the unnecessary words 'the subgroup of'
- changed the long words 'deteriorates' and 'opportunity' to the shorter words 'gets worse' and 'chance'
- split the second sentence into two
- used the verbs 'to prevent' and 'need' instead of the deverbal nouns 'prevention' and 'a need'
- used the first person 'us' and 'We'
- added in a brief explanation of the technical jargon 'preventive programmes'.

EXAMPLE 7

Original sentence: 'This time last year, we were busy making preparations for the opening of the Day Care Unit. It has now been operational since last Easter, taking more patients and with more facilities in a "made-to-measure" environment.'

Plain sentence: 'This time last year, we were busy preparing for the opening of the Day Care Unit, where patients living at home can come for the day. It has now been open since Easter, taking more patients and with more facilities adapted to suit individual needs.'

What I did: In Chapter 7, I changed the word 'operational' to 'open', arguing that it did not matter that this was similar to the word 'opening' already used in the previous sentence. I have then:

- deleted the unnecessary word 'last' in 'since last Easter'
- changed the buzz phrase 'in a "made-to-measure" environment' to 'adapted to suit individual needs'
- changed the deverbal noun 'preparations' to the verb 'preparing'
- added in a brief explanation of the technical jargon 'Day Care Unit'.

EXAMPLE 8

Original sentence: 'It was noted that cash from the management underspend has been identified to support the plan but there was concern that if there were no monies available in the future, interest would drop and the plan would not be delivered.'

Plain sentence: 'We have identified cash from the management underspend (money we expected to spend on management but have saved) to support the plan. But we are concerned that if there is no money available in the future, interest will drop and we will not achieve the plan.'

What I did: In Chapter 7, I split this long sentence into two. I have then:

- deleted the useless words 'It was noted that'
- changed the old-fashioned, legal-sounding 'monies' to the everyday 'money'
- changed the buzz word 'deliver' (which many members of the public think of as what the Royal Mail does) to 'achieve'
- used the active verbs 'have identified' and 'would not achieve' instead of the passive 'was identified' and 'would not be delivered'
- used the first person 'We'
- added in a brief explanation of the technical jargon 'management underspend'.

EXAMPLE 9

Original sentence: 'Directors are asked to note the current position, be aware that there are likely to be further developments in the situation in coming months and endorse the action taken so far to address our paramount concern which is the health and well being of local residents.'

Plain sentence: 'Directors are asked to:

- note the position
- be aware that the situation is likely to develop further in coming months
- support the action taken so far to tackle our main concern, the health and well being of local residents.'

What I did: In Chapter 7, I rearranged the list of items as bullet points. I have then:

- got rid of the useless words 'current' and 'which is'
- changed the unfamiliar words 'endorse', 'address' and 'paramount' to the more usual 'support', 'tackle' and 'main'
- used the verb 'to develop' instead of the deverbal noun 'developments'.

I have left the passive 'are asked', because:

- the agent is obvious (the writer of the board paper)
- starting the sentence with the recipient ('Directors' – who are the readers) draws the audience's attention to the fact that they are being asked to do something.

EXAMPLE 1O

Original sentence: 'Jane was gladdened by the improvement the children had shown even after such a relatively short space of time.'
Plain sentence: 'Jane was pleased by how much the children had improved so fast.'
What I did: In Chapter 7, I changed the deverbal noun 'improvement' to the verb 'had improved'. I have then:

- changed the unusual word 'gladdened' to the more familiar 'pleased'
- simplified the long phrase 'even after such a relatively short space of time' to the much shorter 'so fast'.

EXAMPLE 11

Original sentence: 'The Trust is undertaking a thorough review of its activities to ensure compliance with existing and forthcoming provision in the Disability Discrimination Act.'
Plain sentence: 'We are thoroughly reviewing our activities to make sure we comply with the Disability Discrimination Act (which gives new rights to disabled people), now and in the future.'
What I did: In Chapter 7, I changed the deverbal nouns 'review', 'compliance' and 'provision' to the verbs 'is reviewing', 'complies' and 'provides for'. I have then:

- deleted the useless words 'what' and 'provides for'

- changed 'ensure' to 'make sure'
- used the first person 'We' and 'our'
- added in a brief explanation of the technical jargon 'Disability Discrimination Act'.

EXAMPLE 12

Original sentence: 'A mind-mapping exercise will be undertaken by the whole group on trends around clinical governance, to share current reality and provide data for dialogue.'

Plain sentence: 'The whole group will do a mind-mapping exercise (a way of noting down related ideas and questions). They will look at trends in clinical governance (a system for making sure clinical services are up to scratch). This will help them to swap views on what is happening, and will provide material for discussion.'

What I did: In Chapter 7, I changed the passive verb 'will be undertaken' to the active 'will undertake'. I have then:

- changed the long word 'undertake' to the simpler 'do'
- simplified the buzz phrases 'to share current reality and provide data for dialogue' to 'swap views on what is happening' and 'provide material for discussion'
- changed the buzz word 'around' to the more usual 'in'. ('Around' has become hugely popular in NHS management in recent years. We no longer work on things, or discuss things – we 'do work around', and discuss 'issues around' them)
- added in a brief explanation of the technical jargon 'mind-mapping' and 'clinical governance'. Doing this made the sentence over 40 words, which was too long, so I split it into three.

EXAMPLE 13

Original sentence: 'As we enter the third millennium, the challenge that is faced by us all is to demonstrate that the co-ordinated efforts of local organisations and local people can bring greater improvements in health and well being than if we work alone.'

Plain sentence: 'We all now face a challenge. As local organisations and people, we must show that we can improve health and well being more by working together than by working alone.'

What I did: In Chapter 7, I changed the passive verb 'is faced' to the active 'face'. I have then:

- deleted the second 'local', which is not needed
- changed the phrase 'As we enter the third millennium' to 'now' (Phrases like this seem to be the millennial equivalent of the politicians' old favourite, 'at this moment in time'!)
- changed the long word 'demonstrate' to the shorter and more familiar 'show'
- replaced the words 'co-ordinated efforts' with the more everyday 'working together'
- split the sentence into two to keep down the average sentence length
- used the verb 'improve' in place of the deverbal noun 'improvements'
- added in an extra 'we' to put the whole sentence in the first person.

EXAMPLE 14

Original sentence: 'The Trust recognises the importance of keeping our patients and purchasers fully informed of developments within the organisation and within the NHS nationally.'
Plain sentence: 'We think it is important to keep you up to date with what is going on in our organisation and in the NHS nationally.'
What I did: In Chapter 7, I put the sentence into the first and second person, changing 'The Trust' and 'our patients and purchasers' to the first person 'we' and second person 'you'. I have then:

- got rid of the useless second 'within'
- simplified 'recognise the importance', 'informed', 'developments' and 'within' to 'think it is important', 'up to date', 'what is going on' and 'in'.

EXAMPLE 15

Original sentence: 'The strategy will not lead to a diminution of existing core service provision.'
Plain sentence: 'The strategy will safeguard the core services (important, basic services needed in all areas) that we now provide.'
What I did: In Chapter 7, I changed the sentence from negative to positive. I have then:

- changed the deverbal noun 'provision' to the verb 'provide'
- introduced the first person 'we'
- changed 'existing' to 'now', as this is simpler and fits better with the new sentence
- added in a brief explanation of the technical jargon 'core services'.

EXAMPLE 16

Original sentence: 'These quality improvements have not been gained lightly, but by the dedication, commitment, hard work and teamwork of all staff. Not satisfied to rest on its laurels, however, the Trust is now looking towards the European Foundation of Quality Management model as a target for the future.'

Plain sentence: 'We have improved quality through hard work, by the dedication, commitment and teamwork of all staff. Keen to improve further, however, we are now looking towards the European Foundation of Quality Management model as a target for the future. This is a way of making sure that we provide high quality services, in particular through measuring clinical results.'

What I did: In Chapter 7, I changed the negatives to positives. I have then:

- changed the deverbal noun 'improvements' to the verb 'have improved'
- put both sentences into the first person 'we'
- added an explanation of the technical jargon 'European Foundation of Quality Management model'. Because it was hard to do this in just a few words, I have put it in a short extra sentence.

REFERENCE

1   North West Anglia Health Authority (1988) *The Health of Wisbech: communications and information questionnaire carried out by the Public Engagement Group: report of findings*. North West Anglia Health Authority, Peterborough.

CHAPTER 9

TESTING AND REVISING YOUR PLAIN DOCUMENT

Few people can sit down and write a perfect document straight off. One of the advantages of writing over spontaneous speech is that you get a chance to revise what you say, and how you say it, before it reaches your audience.

At first, you might 'translate' a jargon-ridden draft into plain language, rather than write it in plain English straight away. But even once you have cut out the translating stage, revising what you have written is a natural part of producing a document.

One of the core principles of plain language, as mentioned in Chapter 6, is testing communications on the target audience. This testing is an integral part of the revising stage. Without it, you would not know in what ways you needed to revise your document.

AREAS TO TEST

Testing of documents commonly seeks to measure the audience's:

- understanding of the document
- speed of reading the document
- liking for the document.

METHODS OF TESTING

Figure 8.1 showed a simple view of the writing process, with one box labelled 'test and revise'. But a more detailed look at this stage would show that it is cyclic (*see* Figure 9.1).

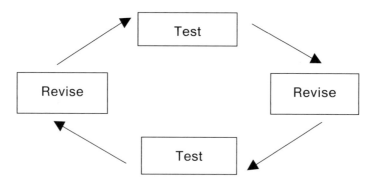

Figure 9.1   A close-up of the testing and revising stage.

Whether you want (and have the chance) to test and revise a document twice (or even more) will depend on:

- the importance of the document – and so how thoroughly you wish to test it
- the time available – both the deadline for finishing the document, and how much work time you or your team can afford to spend on testing
- the budget available.

These factors will affect your choice of methods of testing, which include:

- checking the document yourself, using the plain language guidelines, and your own knowledge and experience
- using text-editing software and readability formulae
- getting colleagues to comment
- commissioning plain English experts to check the document
- testing on the real audience.

The following sections discuss each of these methods.

Checking the text yourself

Once you have produced a reasonable draft of a document, the usual first stage is to check it yourself. You may find it useful to refer to plain language guidelines before you start or as you check. Ask yourself: does the text get your message across to the audience? Only make changes that help it do this better, otherwise you are not really improving the text, and so are wasting time.

This type of testing is important (and you should always make time to do it, even if only quickly). But it is not enough, because it is hard to look at your own work objectively. It has the advantages, however, of having no cost (apart from your time) and being quick (since you are not depending on anyone else's cooperation).

Using text-editing software and readability formulae

Another method that is quick and free, and is more objective but does not rely on other people, is using text-editing software. Grammar checkers that are integral to word-processing packages will pick up on a number of areas where you have not followed plain language guidelines. Remember, however, that they are undiscriminating. For example, they will suggest getting rid of all passive verbs, some of which you may have used with good reason. There are more sophisticated versions that are specifically tailored to plain English (such as Stylewriter–the Plain English Editor, mentioned in Chapter 7).

After checking your document, most text-editing programs show a number of readability statistics, including the results of applying readability formulae. These formulae claim to be able to work out how hard a text is to read, and give their results as numerical scores. These scores are most often expressed as American grade levels. You can convert them to British reading ages by adding five to the grade level score.

When writing for the general public, you should aim for a maximum reading age of 15 (so an American grade level of 10). Remember that if you have to produce a document for a mixed audience, aim it at the least informed (*see* Chapter 6). Where the motivation to read a document is likely to be low, text should be simpler than people are capable of reading.

There are many different readability formulae. Two of the most popular are the Flesch–Kincaid Grade Level and the Gunning Fog Index. If you use the grammar checker in Microsoft Word, the readability statistics it gives at the end include the Flesch–Kincaid Grade Level. This readability formula is therefore easy to use if you write using a word processor. (Remember that if you find it annoying to wade through the full grammar check just to get to your readability statistics, you can usually turn off all grammar check elements except 'show readability statistics'.)

The Flesch–Kincaid Grade Level is the US Department of Defense standard test, and many US government departments use it to test their documents. Box 9.1 shows how the formula works.

Box 9.1: How the Flesch-Kincaid Grade Level formula works

1 Works out the average sentence length by dividing the number of words by the number of sentences
2 Works out the average number of syllables per word by dividing the number of syllables by the number of words
3 Applies the following formula to arrive at the American grade level:
   (Average sentence length × 0.39) + (average number of syllables per word × 11.8) − 15.59
   (Remember that you can convert the American grade level to the British reading age by adding five to this final score.)

This readability formula is less easy to use when writing manually. An easier version is the Gunning Fog Index, invented by Robert Gunning, a pioneer in business communications (*see* Box 9.2).

Box 9.2: How to work out the Gunning Fog Index for your text

1 Take a passage of around 100 words from your text. This should consist of complete sentences only – so do not worry if the sample has slightly more or fewer than 100 words
2 Work out the average sentence length by dividing the number of words by the number of sentences
3 Count the number of words with three or more syllables, but excluding:

   • words that start with capital letters
   • words that are over three syllables because they have had '-ing', '-ed' or '-es' added on the end
   • words that combine two easy words, for example 'anti-smoking' and 'photocopy'.

   This gives you the percentage of hard words.

---

4 Add together the average sentence length and the number of hard words, and multiply the total by 0.4. The result is the lowest American grade level that could easily read the text.
(Remember that you can convert the American grade level to British reading age by adding five to this final score.)

Example
This example uses the extract from a health improvement programme, made plain in Chapter 7, plus the rest of the paragraph it was taken from. I have scored both the original and plain versions, to give two examples of using the Gunning Fog Index, and to show how making text plain generally improves its score

Working out the Gunning Fog score for the original version

Step 1: Take a passage of around 100 words, including whole sentences only
'As we enter the third millennium the challenge that is faced by us all is to demonstrate that the co-ordinated efforts of local organisations and local people can bring greater improvements in health and well being than if we work alone. The delivery of a range of preventative, treatment and care services, managed efficiently and effectively, is important to local people. Equally important is that these services are accessible to all. However, if we are to bring about a lasting improvement in health and well being, we also need to tackle the root causes of ill health.'

Step 2: Work out the average sentence length by dividing the number of words by the number of sentences
97 (number of words) ÷ 4 (number of sentences) = 24.25 (average sentence length)

Step 3: Count the number of words with three or more syllables, to give you the percentage of hard words
Number of words with three or more syllables = 13

Step 4: Add together the average sentence length and the number of hard words, and multiply the total by 0.4
24.25 (average sentence length) + 13 (number of hard words) = 37.25
37.25 × 0.4 = 14.9

The lowest American grade level that could easily read the text is 14.9. Adding five to this gives you the British reading age: 19.9 – too high for text aimed at the general public

Working out the Gunning Fog score for the plain version

Step 1: Take a passage of around 100 words, including whole sentences only
'We all now face a challenge. As local organisations and people, we must show that we can improve health and well being more by working together than by working alone. Providing a range of well managed services to prevent and treat ill health, and care for people with health problems, is important to local people. It is just as important that these services are easy for everyone to use. But if we want to improve health and well being for good, we also need to tackle the root causes of ill health.'

Step 2: Work out the average sentence length by dividing the number of words by the number of sentences
92 (number of words) ÷ 5 (number of sentences) = 18.4 (average sentence length)

Step 3: Count the number of words with three or more syllables, to give you the percentage of hard words
Number of words with three or more syllables = 4

Step 4: Add together the average sentence length and the number of hard words, and multiply the total by 0.4
18.4 (average sentence length) + 4 (number of hard words) = 22.4
22.4 × 0.4 = 9.0

The lowest American grade level that could easily read the text is 9.0. Adding five to this gives you the British reading age – 14.

Microsoft Word also gives you a second readability score – the Flesch Reading Ease score. This gives a score from 0 to 100 (with higher scores representing greater reading ease), rather than a grade level score. This makes it less useful in organisations where some people draft documents on word processors and others manually, as you cannot compare the results with those of the Gunning Fog Index as easily. However, Table 9.1 gives an approximate idea of how the Flesch Reading Ease equates to grade level scores.

Readability formulae are often criticised for not predicting the true reading ease of a piece of text, for a number of reasons. First, they look only at language. They cannot take into account other important elements of the plain language approach such as:

• how interesting the text is to the reader

Table 9.1:   How the Flesch Reading Ease equates to grade level scores[1]

Flesch Reading Ease score	Equivalent American grade level score (British reading age in brackets)
90–100	5th grade (British reading age 10)
80–90	6th grade (British reading age 11)
70–80	7th grade (British reading age 12)
60–70	8–9th grade (British reading age 13–14)
50–60	10–12th grade (British reading age 15–17)
30–50	13–16th grade (British reading age 18–21)
0–30	College graduate

- the writer's attitude, and how this makes people feel when they read the text
- how well structured the document is (including how easy graphics are to understand)
- how clear the layout and design are.

Second, the formulae measure language in a rather crude way (usually by looking at the length of sentences and proportion of difficult words). They tend to ignore other important elements of language (for example, the use of active verbs, the first and second person, and positive statements).

Third, although there is much research evidence to show that generally we understand more and faster when words and sentences are short and simple, it is true that:

- long words and sentences are not always difficult to understand For example, readability formulae cannot take into account whether or not you have explained a difficult word. Using technical jargon in a document, with a simple explanation, is more in keeping with the plain language principle of empowering people than getting rid of it altogether. Yet taking this approach may often give you a less good readability score
- short words and sentences are not always easy to understand. This is truer for certain types of writing, for example poetry and text on mathematics. These often use a naturally terse and condensed style. It applies less to the general information-giving documents that NHS communicators are likely to be writing.

In summary, readability formulae are useful, so long as we remember their limitations and do not try to assign too grand a meaning to their results.

Use them for analysing objectively what you have already written, as a broad indicator of the extent to which you have followed the guidelines on writing plainly. They are also good for comparing different documents, or different versions of the same document. If line managers, and committees or other groups, want to amend your work, the formulae can show whether they really are making it plainer or not.

GETTING COLLEAGUES TO COMMENT

In common with text-editing software, asking colleagues to check your work for plainness has the advantage of being more objective than checking it yourself. It has the advantage over text-editing software of bringing a human viewpoint to testing. A study compared the changes suggested by text-editing software and colleagues' comments. This showed that text-editing programs were more thorough and systematic than colleagues. But colleagues offered comments on a broader range of aspects of a document's plainness.[1]

One potential disadvantage of asking colleagues to comment is that they may not be the target audience for your document. Their feedback may not therefore improve the text for the real audience. The relative power of the writer and person commenting can affect this. For example, staff may feel constrained in commenting on bosses' writing. Bosses may make a lot of minor changes in staff members' writing, as a way of asserting authority.

One of the areas where colleagues' feedback on documents intended for the general public is particularly unreliable is whether or not they sound condescending. NHS communicators seem prone to worry that plain language sounds condescending when the real audience does not find it so, appreciating the clear presentation (*see*, for example, Box 4.2).

COMMISSIONING PLAIN ENGLISH EXPERTS

Although they would not claim to be a substitute for testing on the real audience, plain English consultants (such as those listed in Box 2.2) are expert in how readable a document is likely to be for the real audience.

Although using an external organisation may mean you have to allow a little more time for testing the document, many consultants are able to turn work round within a few days (although sometimes at a premium price).

Plain language organisations often offer kitemarking schemes, where they will accredit a particular document as written in plain language. You can then include a logo on it showing this. Some plain language organisations charge a flat-rate fee per document, based on its length, while others vary their fee depending on how much editing work is needed to bring the document up to scratch. The complete process can be expensive and so is probably best suited to high-profile documents.

Another possibility is to include in your plain language training (*see* Chapter 2) in-depth training for a small number of people who can then act as an in-house editorial team.

TESTING ON THE REAL AUDIENCE

There is no substitute for testing documents on the real audience, provided you have the time and money to do this. You can use various techniques, some of which demand a lot of time, expertise and special tools. However, research has shown that such testing does not need to be hugely elaborate or to involve quantitative data that are statistically watertight. People who are not specifically trained in research methods can test a document effectively using basic qualitative methods.[2] For example, you can use interviews, group discussions, observations or questionnaire surveys to test how easily your audience understands the document.

With the increased emphasis on encouraging increased public, patient and staff involvement, your organisation will already:

- have in place groups that you could test documents on (for example, staff focus groups, user groups and health panels). You can even use family and friends (for testing a document intended for the general public), or colleagues (for one intended for NHS staff). This makes the process quicker and easier, but make sure that the people you test your document on are reasonably representative of the rest of the audience. For example, if you check a document for the general public with people who are all university graduates, you will not get representative feedback
- be familiar with the possible methods of gathering people's views, such as face-to-face interviews, telephone interviewing and postal questionnaires.

Much of the good practice that you already know is just as relevant to testing documents, while other guidelines are more specific (*see* Box 9.3).

Box 9.3: Good practice guidelines on testing documents with real audiences

General good practice on involving the public, patients and staff

- Be specific about what you ask people to do. If you raise expectations beyond what is realistic, you may end up with a lot of general or detailed comments on areas that you may not want or be able to change anyway. For example, if your message is an unpopular one (such as reducing services), you could end up with a discussion of this rather than of the clarity of the document. Many people also enjoy being picky about written language, arguing about small points of style that do not affect how easily the document is understood

- Make sure that people are not out of pocket as a result of getting involved in your testing
- If you do not act on people's suggestions, make sure you have a good reason, and explain this
- Remember to thank people, perhaps acknowledge their contribution in the document (if they would like you to), and give them feedback on how their involvement helped to improve the document

Good practice specific to the testing of documents

- When testing the audience's understanding of the document, ask them to read it once only. Documents written in plain language should be easy to understand on the first reading. In real life, people will not normally bother to read again a document that is not
- If testing a document on a group of people who are all present in the same place at the same time, make it clear that you are testing the document, not them. For example, when testing the audience's understanding of the document, try to make people feel comfortable about speaking out about difficulties without feeling that they are being stupid. Make it clear that your organisation accepts responsibility for how easy or difficult the document is to understand. One way of getting more honest feedback can be to ask people to point out what difficulties they think others (rather than they themselves) might have in understanding the document. You could also use (either instead of, or as well as, a group discussion) a questionnaire to be completed and handed in. This gives people a chance to record any difficulties in a more private way

Similarly, when testing the audience's speed of reading the document, ask them:

- to read at a speed that is natural and comfortable to them, not to compete with others to finish first
- to write down (rather than say) how long they took to read it
- not to make a display of finishing (such as putting down pens obviously or shuffling papers)

Choosing what method(s) to use

Table 9.2 summarises the methods of testing discussed above, and rates them in terms of thoroughness, speed of turn-around possible, demand on staff time and cost (other than that of staff time). This should help you select a method right for your particular document and circumstances.

Table 9.2: Pros and cons of different methods of testing a document for plainness

Method	Thorough-ness	Speed of turn-around possible	Demand on staff time	Cost
Checking yourself	✓	✓✓✓✓	✓✓✓✓	✓✓✓✓
Using readability formulae	✓✓	✓✓✓✓	✓✓✓✓	✓✓✓✓
Getting colleagues to comment	✓✓	✓✓✓	✓✓	✓✓✓✓
Commissioning plain English experts	✓✓✓	✓✓	✓✓✓	✓
Testing on the real audience	✓✓✓✓	✓	✓	✓

✓✓✓✓ = best (i.e. thorough, fast turn-around, low demand on staff time and low cost)

✓ = least good (i.e. least thorough, slow turn-around, high demand on staff time and high cost)

You do not need to use just one method. You can combine these to good effect.

- You could use readability formulae to get a document to a reasonable level of plainness before getting it checked by a plain language expert. This is likely to bring down the cost of using the expert, through reducing the number of changes needed at that stage.
- You could use colleagues' comments to improve a document intended for the general public before testing it on the real audience. This may reduce the time involved in, and cost of, the latter.

It is not feasible to put most documents that you produce through the more thorough forms of testing. Most of us churn out several letters, memos and papers every day, and we are lucky to get time even to check them over quickly ourselves. Do try, however, to use the more thorough forms of testing sometimes. Remember that anything is better than nothing, in terms of both:

- the proportion of documents you test at all – so if you test just one document every few months, you will learn useful lessons on communicating plainly that you can then apply to other documents you do not have time to test. You can even incorporate these lessons into the organisation's style guide, as guidelines to help others improve their documents more quickly and easily
- how thoroughly you test each document – so if you do not have time to use a readability formula on a letter, check it yourself using the plain language guidelines; or if you do not have time to test an annual report on the real audience, get a plain English expert to have a look.

Remember too that testing important documents is an investment; the cost of whatever testing is done should pay for itself many times over, in the benefits described in Chapter 3.

Finally, even once you have finished whatever testing you have decided to do, and your document is complete, make it easy for people reading the final, published version to comment and ask questions. For example, include a tear-off form for readers to jot down their comments on and send in. And tell people who they can contact, and where, with any queries.

REFERENCES

1   Hartley J (1994) *Designing Instructional Text* (3e). Kogan Page, London.
2   Kempson E and Moore N (1994) *Designing Public Documents: a review of research*. Policy Studies Institute, London.

CHAPTER 10

COMMUNICATING IN SPEECH AND OTHER SPECIAL CIRCUMSTANCES

Plain language experts tend to advise on writing paper-based documents, in English, for a general readership. It is true that most management information is disseminated in this way, to this audience. But this approach is rather narrow, given that:

- spoken language – both planned and spontaneous – can be jargon ridden too
- documents are increasingly being published electronically rather than on paper, for example through emails and on websites
- many NHS organisations need to communicate with people who do not speak English, or whose first language is not English
- the audience for an NHS communication may have other special needs (such as being blind or partially sighted).

In fact, most of the plain language guidelines are relevant to all these types of communication. Following the standard guidelines will make a communication using any medium easier for any target audience to understand. When communicating in media other than paper-based writing, or with audiences other than the general public, it is, however, useful to be aware of any:

- recommended changes to the standard guidelines
- additional guidelines
- sources of more detailed information.

These can help you tailor your communication more finely to the medium and the target audience and are described in this chapter.

COMMUNICATING IN SPEECH

There are two different types of spoken communication:

- planned – such as speeches, presentations, video commentaries, and audio tape recordings
- spontaneous.

This division may not be clear-cut. For example, a planned presentation may lead to a question-and-answer session in which responses are, inevitably, spontaneous. In the same way, there may be an overlap with written communications. For example, in a presentation, you may use written slides or provide a written handout.

Figure 10.1 illustrates the processes of producing written, planned spoken and spontaneous spoken communications, showing the key differences between these. You can see that there are far fewer differences between written and planned spoken communications than there are between written and spontaneous spoken ones. Even so, the differences from written communications have a number of important implications.

PLANNING YOUR PLAIN SPOKEN COMMUNICATION

In spontaneous speech, the much shorter time available for planning means you have to think on your feet rather than having time to work steadily through the guidelines. Being familiar with the guidelines will help, however, as setting a brief for and structuring (albeit quickly) what you are about to say will make your speaking plainer.

The speed required to do this clearly makes it difficult, but it will get easier with practice.

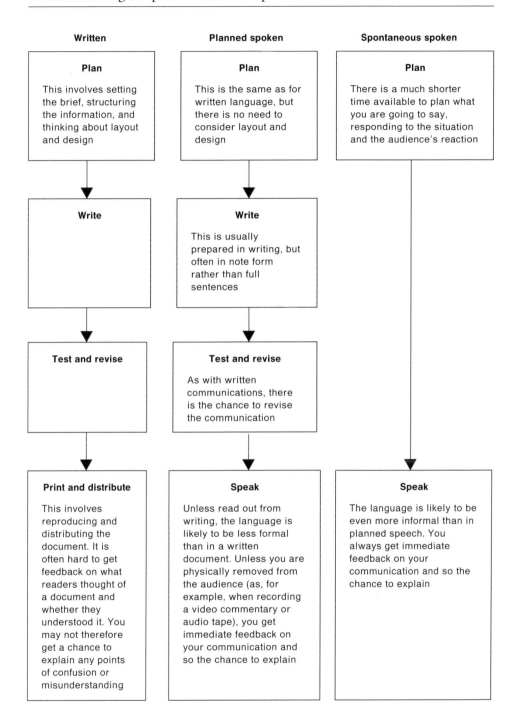

Figure 10.1 The processes of producing written, planned spoken and spontaneous spoken communications.

SPEAKING PLAINLY

In speech (particularly spontaneous), following many of the guidelines on using plain words, phrases and sentences comes relatively naturally, for various reasons, such as:

- the language we use in speech is generally less formal
- having less time to plan and revise the communication makes sentence structures less complex
- more often than not you are addressing the listeners directly, which makes them seem less removed and so encourages a less formal style. Plain language experts often advise that when writing, you should imagine the reader sitting opposite you.

However, jargon may still creep in. Buzz words, gobbledegook words and phrases, and technical jargon do appear in speech. Gobbledegook structures are less common in speech, but can occasionally occur when it is planned and the speaker is not face to face with the audience (such as in a video commentary or on an audio tape).

In planned speech, the testing and revising stage should eliminate negative jargon use, but in spontaneous speech there is no such stage. The two main ways of tackling this are:

- avoiding it in the first place, by trying to bear in mind constantly the audience you are talking to. I find it useful to imagine a mental 'sieve', through which I visualise passing what I am about to say, filtering out inappropriate jargon. This is really just the same mechanism that stops us 'putting our foot in it' through thinking before we speak
- putting it right when it does slip through, by encouraging the audience to feel free to speak up if they do not understand anything you say. Chapter 9 includes some tips on doing this. In important public meetings, it can also be useful to ask someone assertive from outside the NHS (for example, a journalist or television presenter) to come along and challenge any words or phrases they do not understand. You are immediately alerted to explain what you mean.

As in written communications, explain technical jargon to audiences who are not familiar with it, as you mention it. You may like to back this up with a written sheet of explanations for listeners to refer to. So as not to distract listeners from listening to you, give this out after you have finished speaking, for them to refer to later.

TESTING AND REVISING YOUR PLAIN COMMUNICATION

Many of the tips given under the plain language guidelines rely on there being time to revise your communication, which you do not have the chance to do in spontaneous speech. But you can reflect on your spoken language and use the tips to improve the plainness of your language in the future. It can be useful to record yourself in spontaneous speech, so you are not relying on your own or other people's memory of what you said, and so you can be more objective about your performance. You can then check this yourself later against the plain language guidelines.

You can also ask your audience for feedback on how plain they have found your spoken communication, possibly using the methods described in Chapter 9. Even if this is not feasible, one advantage of speaking over writing is that you can see how the audience reacts to your communication. As you speak, you will get clues (through comments, questions and body language) on how well the audience is following what you are saying.

COMMUNICATING THROUGH ELECTRONIC MEDIA

If you follow the standard guidelines, your electronic text will undoubtedly become more readable. There are, however, some additional considerations to bear in mind if you are writing text for electronic media, for example websites. Box 10.1 summarises these.

Box 10.1: Additional considerations when writing electronic text

Structure
- You cannot flick through an electronic document as easily as a paper-based one, and can only ever see part of it at any time. This makes it harder to get an overall idea of its structure and to work out where you are in relation to the document as a whole. It is therefore particularly important to plan a clear structure

Layout and design
- Page size is smaller, as a normal-sized screen holds less than an A4 page. Page orientation is also different, a screen being landscape shaped (wider than it is long) and a page usually portrait shaped (the opposite). You therefore need to think about the shape and size of any graphics, to make sure that readers can see the whole thing at once

- There are extra variables in electronic media beyond those in paper-based ones, for example flicker, glare and resolution. It may also be more tempting to use colour, as you are not dependent on having a colour printer or photocopier (and the associated larger budget) to reproduce the document

Writing
- People tend to scan web pages, picking out words and sentences, rather than reading them word for word. Following the standard plain language guidelines will make scanning easier, but there are extra things you can do to make a website more user friendly. For example, you can highlight key words and use fewer words than in conventional writing

Box 10.2 contains a list of sources of detailed advice on communicating through electronic media.

Box 10.2: Communicating using electronic media: further information

Book
Hartley J (1994) *Designing Instructional Text* (3e). Kogan Page, London. (See chapter on 'Designing electronic text')

Guidelines
The NHS Identity Guidelines (available at http://www.dihnet.org.uk/nhsidentity/index.htm) give guidance on designing NHS websites, and include a 'web-safe colour palette'.
    Other advice and links are available through the NHS Executive's Guidance on providing online public information about local healthcare services (available at http://www.doh.gov.uk/nhsexipu/whatnew/eguide.html).

Websites
- http://www.ibm.com/ibm/easy/
- http://www.microsoft.com/enable/
- http://hubel.sfasu.edu/research/survreslts.html
- http://www.useit.com/alertbox/9710a.html
- http://www.wordsmyth.com/webtips.html

Several of these provide useful links to other related sites.

COMMUNICATING WITH AUDIENCES WITH SPECIAL NEEDS

Most NHS communications are intended for general audiences, but you may sometimes want to communicate with an audience with special needs, for example:

- people who are blind or partially sighted
- people who are hard of hearing
- older people
- people who have reading and writing difficulties
- people whose first language is not English.

Again, following the standard guidelines will make communications more accessible to all these groups. However, there is specialist guidance on making them even more so.

PEOPLE WHO ARE BLIND OR PARTIALLY SIGHTED

People who are blind or partially sighted may have problems reading written communications prepared for a general audience.

In fact, only 20% of people who are registered blind are completely blind and so need Braille transcriptions or tape recordings of written text.[1] The standard plain language guidelines will in any case make communications using both these special media more easily understandable.

Many of the remaining 80% of people registered blind can read large print, using plain fonts of at least size 14. There are no advantages in using

---

Box 10.3: Communicating with people who are blind or partially sighted: further information

- Hartley J (1994) *Designing Instructional Text* (3e). Kogan Page, London. (See chapter on 'Text design for the visually impaired')
- Royal National Institute for the Blind (RNIB) *'See it Right' Information Pack*. RNIB, London.

The RNIB also provides information on producing Braille documents, tape recordings and electronic text for people with sight loss. You can contact them at: RNIB, 224 Great Portland Street, London W1N 6AA (tel: 020 7388 1266; fax: 020 7388 2034) email: cservices@rnib.org.uk; website: http://www.rnib.org.uk

text any larger than font size 20.[2] Again, the standard guidelines will improve the readability of such larger print documents.

Box 10.3 gives details of specialist information on communicating with people who are blind or partially sighted.

PEOPLE WHO ARE HARD OF HEARING

People who were born deaf or became deaf when very young are likely to have a much smaller vocabulary than those who can hear.[3] For this reason, using familiar words is particularly important.

OLDER PEOPLE

Some older people may also have eyesight problems that make it difficult for them to read written communications intended for a general audience. In addition, people's working memory often declines. This means that they can hold less information in the short term, for use in ongoing tasks. This can affect how readily they understand both written and spoken communications.

Although the standard guidelines will help, you need to pay attention to print size, using plain font sizes of at least size 12. You should also pay special attention to structure and layout, making these reflect the sense of the communication as clearly as possible. It will also help people with reduced working memory if you adapt the language, using shorter and less complex sentences.

Box 10.4 gives details of a source of specialist guidance on communicating with older people.

Box 10.4: Communicating with older people

Hartley J (1994) *Designing Instructional Text* (3e). Kogan Page, London. (See chapter on 'Instructional text and older readers'. This contains a list of suggested further reading)

PEOPLE WITH READING AND WRITING DIFFICULTIES

There are around 5.5 million people in the UK who have reading and writing difficulties. Only a small number of these cannot read at all, but many find it hard to read text prepared for a general audience.[4]

Following the standard guidelines for communicating in plain language will help these people. As with older people, pay particular attention to structure and layout, and use shorter and less complex sentences. But avoid using larger font sizes than you would use for a general audience. So long as the font is clear, making it larger will not help. Doing so is like repeating the same thing more loudly to a foreigner who has not understood you.

Box 10.5 lists sources of advice on communicating with people who have difficulties with reading and writing.

Box 10.5: Communicating with people who have difficulties with reading and writing

The Basic Skills Agency *Making Reading Easier* (information leaflet). The Basic Skills Agency, London.

The Basic Skills Agency publishes a range of material for and about people who have reading and writing difficulties. You can contact them at: The Basic Skills Agency, Admail 524, London WC1A 1BR (tel: 0870 600 2400; fax: 0870 600 2401) email: enquiries@basic-skills.co.uk; website: http://www.basic-skills.co.uk

---

PEOPLE FROM ETHNIC MINORITIES

Following the standard guidelines for communicating in plain language will make people whose first language is not English much more likely to understand your communication than if you write it in jargon-ridden language.

As Box 3.1 showed, the plain language movement is not restricted to the English-speaking world. Although the plain language guidelines presented in this book are intended to apply specifically to English, many of them may be relevant to communications in other languages. For example, a range of different fonts are available for Asian, Cyrillic and other alphabets, some of which will be clearer than others.

There may also be other plain language guidelines specially designed for a particular language. If you are producing communications in other languages, ask the people you would normally use to translate or interpret and design documents in these languages for advice on this.

Cultural differences may also cause problems in communicating clearly with people whose first language is not English. These differences may mean they interpret parts of a communication quite differently from the way native English speakers would. For example, thought patterns, and so the organisation of written text, vary considerably between different languages.

- English usually has a linear structure.
- Semitic and Arabic languages use series of parallel structures.
- Oriental languages have a circular structure.
- Romance languages (i.e. those derived from Latin, such as French, Italian and Spanish) often include many digressions.
- Indic languages use a spiral structure.[3]

Cultural differences can cause particular problems in interpreting graphics. You again need to seek expert advice, and ideally to test the graphics on members of the target audience.

REFERENCES

1   Hartley J (1994) *Designing Instructional Text* (3e). Kogan Page, London.
2   Kempson E and Moore N (1994) *Designing Public Documents: a review of research*. Policy Studies Institute, London.
3   The Basic Skills Agency *Making Reading Easier* (information leaflet). The Basic Skills Agency, London.
4   Royal National Institute for the Blind (RNIB) *'See it Right' Information Pack*. RNIB, London.

AIDS TO NHS JARGON BUSTING

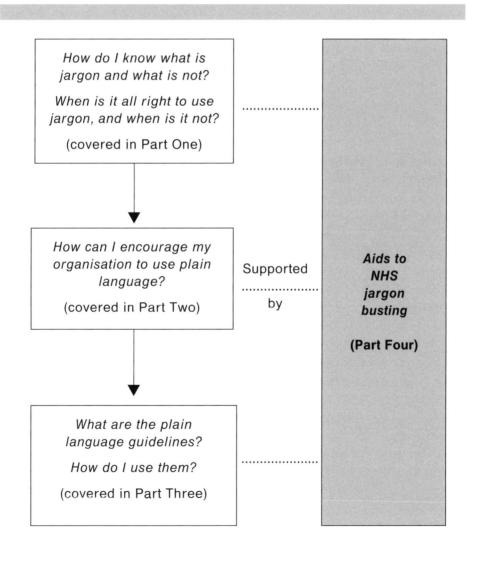

How do I know what is jargon and what is not?

When is it all right to use jargon, and when is it not?

(covered in Part One)

How can I encourage my organisation to use plain language?

(covered in Part Two)

What are the plain language guidelines?

How do I use them?

(covered in Part Three)

Supported

by

Aids to NHS jargon busting

(Part Four)

Examples of NHS Buzz words, with plain English translations

> **Note**
>
> A word of warning – because the meaning of buzz words is often obscure, I have based my plain English 'translations' on what I understand the buzz words to mean. You may not, therefore, agree with my interpretation. Also, I have noted down more than one possible meaning for some buzz words. (This ambiguity is exactly why buzz words are best avoided.)

Buzz word	*Plain English version*
to **access**	to get, get into
to **add value**	to improve, give extra benefit
agenda (for example 'the modernisation agenda')	things we must/need to do to… (for example 'things we must do to make the NHS more modern')

Buzz word	*Plain English version*
animal (as in 'primary care groups are interesting animals')	thing, organisation, person
arena	area, field
around (as in 'to work around', 'issues around')	on, to do with
ballpark (figure)	rough, approximate
to **bottom**	to get to the bottom of, finish
bottom-up	led by staff
to **box** something **off**	to finish something, get something done, sort something out
to **bring up to speed**	to brief, update
to **buy into**	to support
to **capture**	to note
to **cherry pick**	to choose the best
by **close of play**	by the end of the day
someone's **comfort zone**	what someone feels happy with
to **connect with**	to communicate with, understand
cost envelope	available money, budget
to **cover off**	to do
to **deliver**	to do, achieve
deliverables	things we (or you, they, etc.) must/can achieve

Buzz word	*Plain English version*
to **diarise**	to make an appointment
to **dovetail with**	to link in with
driver for change	cause of/reason for change
to **get into bed with**	to work closely with
to **get your ducks in a row**	to get ready, prepare
to **engineer** (a conversation, meeting, etc.)	to arrange, set up
to **factor in**	to include, take account of
to **fast-track**	to do quickly, get done quickly
fit for purpose	suitable
to **flag up**	to point out, raise
to **frame an agenda**	to decide what needs to be done
game plan	plan
to have a **handle on**	to know about, understand
to **have the ball**	to be in control
to **head up**	to lead, be head of
to **helicopter up**	to take an overview, see the broader context
to **hit the ground running**	to start immediately
key player	important person/organisation
to **kick into touch**	to get rid of
level playing field	equal footing
in the **loop**	informed, involved

Buzz word	*Plain English version*
to **map**	to set out how things are
mission statement	aim, goal
movers and shakers	important/influential people
multi-tasking	doing more than one thing
off-line (as in 'to talk about something off-line')	unofficially, outside the meeting/office
to be **on board**	to support
to **parachute** someone **in**	to bring someone in
to **park** something (as in 'let's park that idea')	to leave something for now, put something on one side
to **pick the low-hanging fruit**	to start with the easiest things
to **play back**	to repeat
the **quantum of resource**	the amount of money/people, etc.
a **raft of** (ideas, possibilities, etc.)	many
to **reality-check** something	to see if something is correct/feasible
to **row back on** (a commitment)	to go back on
to **row in the same direction**	to share an aim, want the same result
to **run** something **by** someone	to ask someone what they think of something
to **run with** (an idea, project, etc.)	to go ahead with, put into action, agree with

Buzz word	*Plain English version*
to **scope**	to look into
sexy (as in 'a sexy idea')	attractive, appealing
to **share a vision**	to share an aim, want the same result
to be **signed up to**	to support
to **sing from the same hymn sheet**	to present the same message
to take a **steer from**	to be guided by, follow
to **stitch** someone **into** something	to involve someone in something, keep someone up to date with something
to **task** someone **with** something	to ask someone to do something, give someone the job of doing something
to be a **team player**	to work well with others
to **tease out**	to look at in detail, work out
top-down	led by management
to **touch base with**	to contact, update
to **trawl**	to go through
to **unpack**	to look at in detail, work out
a **window** (as in 'I have a window in my diary next Monday')	some time free, a slot
window of opportunity	opportunity, chance

EXAMPLES OF NHS GOBBLEDEGOOK, WITH PLAIN ENGLISH TRANSLATIONS

Notes

1 Gobbledegook includes not just words and phrases, but whole sentence structures. Because of the almost infinite number of possible structures, this thesaurus cannot give translations of these. Look at the guidelines in Chapter 7, and examples in Chapter 8, on making the structure of your sentences plainer.

2 You may also find it useful to:

- refer to a normal thesaurus (picking out the synonyms that are shortest and most familiar)
- get hold of a copy of the *Plain English Campaign's A-Z Guide of Alternative Words* (available from the Plain English Campaign; *see* Box 2.2 for contact details).

Gobbledegook	*Plain English version*
an **absence of**	no, none
in the **absence of**	without
an **abundance of**	enough, a lot of
to **accentuate**	to stress
accompanying	with
to **accomplish**	to do
in **accordance with**	in line with
to be in **accordance with**	to agree with, follow
accordingly	so
accustomed to	used to
to **acquire**	to get
in **addition to**	as well as
additional	more, extra
to **address**	to think about, tackle, sort out
adequate	enough
ad hoc	for this purpose, one-off
adjacent	next to
in **advance of**	before
advantageous	better, useful
to **advise**	to tell
to **afford an opportunity**	to allow, let

Gobbledegook	*Plain English version*
to **align**	to line up, get in line
to **alleviate**	to ease, reduce
to **allocate**	to share out, give
allocation	share
to **ameliorate**	to improve, help
to **anticipate**	to expect
apparent	clear, obvious
to **apprise**	to tell
appropriate	right
approximately	roughly, about
to **ascertain**	to find out
as of the date of	from, since
to **assemble**	to gather, put together
assistance	help
to **attain**	to reach
to **attempt**	to try
attributable to	due to
axiomatic	obvious
to **bestow**	to give
to **calculate**	to work out
to have the **capability to**	to be able to

Gobbledegook	*Plain English version*
carte blanche	freedom
category	group
circa	about
to **circumvent**	to get round, avoid
in **close proximity**	near
to be **cognisant of**	to know about
to **commence**	to start
commencement	start
competence	skill, ability
to **comply with**	to keep to, meet
component	part
to **comprise**	to be made up of
concept	idea
concerning	about
to **conclude**	to end
concordat	agreement, deal
to **concur**	to agree
in **conjunction with**	with
in **connection with**	about
as a **consequence of**	because
consequently	so

Gobbledegook	*Plain English version*
to **consider**	to think, think about
to give **consideration to**	to think about
to **constitute**	to form, make up
to **contemplate**	to think about
contrary to	against, despite
to **cooperate**	to help
cooperation	help
corroboration	proof
in the **course of**	while, during
to **deem**	to think
to **defer**	to put off, delay
to **demonstrate**	to show
despite the fact that	although
to **determine**	to decide, find out
detrimental	harmful
dialogue	talk, discussion
disbursements	payments
to **disclose**	to show, reveal, tell
to **discontinue**	to stop
discontinuation	end
to **dispose of**	to get rid of

Gobbledegook	*Plain English version*
to **disseminate**	to spread
documentation	papers
due to the fact that	because
to **effect**	to make, bring about
to **elect**	to choose
element	part
to **elucidate**	to explain, make clear
to **emanate from**	to come from
to **enable**	to allow
to **encounter**	to meet with
to **endeavour**	to try
to **enhance**	to improve
to **enquire**	to ask
to **ensue**	to follow
to **ensure**	to make sure
entitlement	right
entrenched	fixed
to **envisage**	to expect, imagine
equitable	fair
equivalent	equal, the same
erroneous	wrong

Gobbledegook	*Plain English version*
to **establish**	to set up, form
in the **event that**	if
excessive	too much
in **excess of**	more than
exclusively	only
to **exhibit**	to show
to **expedite**	to speed up, hurry
expenditure	spending
to **evaluate**	to test, check
to **fabricate**	to make up
to **facilitate**	to help, ease, make easier
factor	reason
feasible	possible
to **formulate**	to plan, come up with
forthwith	now, at once
to **forward**	to send
to **generate**	to give, bring about
on the **grounds that**	because
hitherto	until now
however	but
identical	the same

Gobbledegook	*Plain English version*
to **illustrate**	to show, explain
to **impede**	to block, delay, hold up
to **implement**	to do, carry out
to **imply**	to suggest
inception	start
increment	step, increase
to **indicate**	to show
to **infer that**	to take it that
to **inform**	to say, tell
initial	first
to **initiate**	to start
input	help
to **insert**	to put in
to **inspect**	to look at, check
instance	case
inter alia	among other things
to **jeopardise**	to risk, threaten
legislation	law
in **lieu of**	instead of
location	place
magnitude	size

Gobbledegook	*Plain English version*
to **maintain**	to keep
marginal	small, slight
by **means of**	by
merely	only, just
with the **minimum of delay**	quickly
modification	change
modus operandi	way of working, way of doing things
to **monitor**	to check, watch, keep an eye on
morbidity	ill health, illness, disease
mortality	death, number of deaths, death rate
in the **near future**	soon
negligible	very small
nevertheless	but
to **notify**	to tell
notwithstanding	even though
numerous	many
on **numerous occasions**	often
objective	aim, goal
to **observe**	to see, note
obsolete	out of date

Gobbledegook	*Plain English version*
to **obtain**	to get
to **occur**	to happen
to **operate**	to work, run
to be of the **opinion**	to think
optimum	best, ideal
option	choice
in **order to**	to
outcome	result
out-turn (price, position, etc.)	final, closing
to **participate**	to join in, take part
particulars	details
pending	until
per annum	a year
per capita	per person, a head, each
to **perform**	to do
to **permit**	to let, allow
per se	in itself
to be in **possession of**	to have
at the **present time**	now
prima facie	at first sight
principal	main

Gobbledegook	*Plain English version*
to **prioritise**	to rank
prior to	before
procedure	test, treatment, operation, way of doing things
to **proceed**	to go ahead
to **procure**	to get, buy
pro forma	form
to **progress** something	to move something forward, get on with
to **promulgate**	to make public, spread the word about
proportion	part
provided that	as long as, if
to **purchase**	to buy
to **purport**	to claim
for the **purpose of**	to
to **qualify for**	to be able to get
re	about
to be in **receipt of**	to get
to **receive**	to get
reconfiguration	change
to **reconsider**	to think again about

Gobbledegook	*Plain English version*
to **recover**	to get back
reduction	cut
with **reference to**	about
in **regard to**	about
regarding	about
regulation	rule
to **reimburse**	to repay
to **reiterate**	to repeat, say again
remit	job, task
remittance	payment
remuneration	pay
relating to	about
in **respect of**	about
to **report**	to tell
to **request**	to ask
requirements	needs
resources	money, people, equipment
restriction	limit
to **resume**	to start again
to **retain**	to keep
to **review**	to look at again, check

Gobbledegook	*Plain English version*
to **revise**	to change
to **scrutinise**	to look closely at, check
to **select**	to choose
to **specify**	to say/state clearly
statutory	legal
to **stipulate**	to lay down, insist on
to **submit**	to send, give
subsequently	later
substantial	large
sufficient	enough
to **supplement**	to add to
supplementary	more, extra
to **terminate**	to stop, end
therefore	so
to date	so far
together with	with, and
to **transpire**	to turn out, happen
ultimately	in the end
to **undertake**	to do
to **undertake to**	to agree to
until such time as	until

Gobbledegook	*Plain English version*
utilisation	use
to **utilise**	to use
to **verify**	to prove
with a **view to**	to
virtually	almost
vis-à-vis	about
whereby	by which
zone	area

EXAMPLES OF NHS TECHNICAL JARGON, WITH PLAIN ENGLISH EXPLANATIONS

Notes

1 All examples are of English NHS jargon – for which I apologise to those working in the Northern Irish, Scottish or Welsh NHS. This is because trying to cover all four countries within the space available would have produced a very narrow glossary, containing little more than structural terms. I decided to focus on the English NHS as, being the largest, it is likely to be relevant to more readers.

2 I have chosen technical terms that:

- in my experience, crop up most regularly in common local NHS communications (such as annual reports, websites and public meetings)
- represent a cross-section of the categories of technical jargon listed in Chapter 1.

3 For each technical term, there is:

- a short explanation, for use within your main text
- a longer explanation, for use in a separate glossary (as suggested in Chapter 8).

4 For technical terms that are commonly shortened, I give the acronym or abbreviation. See Chapter 8 for how to deal with acronyms and abbreviations.

5 When using pre-written explanations (whether mine, or from an in-house glossary), you may need to adjust these to fit the context, in terms of content and linguistic structure. For example, exactly what information you include in an explanation, and (for separate glossaries) how detailed you make it, will depend on:

- the purpose of your communication
- the needs of your audience.

My explanations here are fairly general, and you may need to tailor these to your own requirements. For example, in most cases I have not included in my longer explanations the year when each term began (or may cease to exist!), or the reform that introduced them. Although I would expect that most of the time the public does not want or need to know this, it may sometimes be relevant. Similarly, you may need to change the tense of the verbs (that is, whether you are writing in the past, present or future). In the fast-changing NHS, many terms that are current as I write will be past by the time you are reading them! You may also need to change nouns from singular to plural (or vice versa) in the short explanations, to make them slot smoothly into your particular sentence.

Technical jargon	Short explanation	Longer explanation
acute services	hospital services	Acute health services are provided mainly in hospitals. They deal with sudden and more serious health problems. Your GP usually refers you to acute services. You might also refer yourself, for example by going to an accident and emergency (casualty) department

Technical jargon	Short explanation	Longer explanation
benchmarking	comparing the way we do things, to improve quality	Benchmarking compares how one organisation does things with the way that others (which are known to be good) do the same things. This helps the first organisation improve its services and ways of working
care pathway	plan for treating people with a particular health problem	Care pathways are plans that show the steps proven to be important in caring for patients with a particular health problem. They show the progress that you can expect a typical patient to make each day of the treatment. All the local healthcare staff who are involved in treating and caring for patients agree the pathways. For example, doctors, nurses and therapists may be involved
care trust	an organisation providing both health and social care	Care trusts will include health and social services. They may also include other local authority services, such as housing. This will help stop patients from falling into the cracks between services. It will also stop people being left in hospital when they could be safely in their own home. In particular, care trusts will help people who need a range of services, often over a long time. For example, they will help older people and people with mental health problems
case mix	the mixture of health problems, and how severe these are	In one hospital ward, or one GP surgery, there may be patients with a wide range of health problems. These problems may differ in how easy or hard they are to treat. This mixture of health problems, and how severe they are, is called 'case mix'

Technical jargon	Short explanation	Longer explanation
clinical audit	a way for healthcare staff to measure the quality of care	When doctors and other healthcare staff do clinical audit, they look regularly at the quality of care they have provided. This helps them pinpoint good and bad parts of this care, which they can then build on or tackle
clinical directorate	a group of hospital departments, led by one consultant	Many hospitals are organised into clinical directorates. These are groups of departments, led by one consultant. This consultant is responsible to the hospital board for managing the directorate
clinical governance	a system for making sure clinical services are up to scratch	Clinical governance is a national system for making sure clinical services are up to scratch. NHS organisations now have a legal duty to make sure clinical care is of a high quality. NHS chief executives are held to account for the clinical standards within their organisations
Clinical Negligence Scheme for Trusts (CNST)	a scheme that pays the costs of claims for clinical negligence	The Clinical Negligence Scheme for Trusts (CNST) pays the costs of claims for clinical negligence. Trusts pay a subscription to join the CNST, based on their likely level of claims. In return, the CNST meets the costs of claims above a certain amount. This is rather like an insurance policy, where paying the premium covers you for costs above your excess
Commission for Health Improvement (CHI)	the national organisation that checks clinical standards	The Commission for Health Improvement checks clinical standards in every part of the NHS in England and Wales. It does spot checks, and helps NHS organisations that are having problems with clinical quality

Technical jargon	Short explanation	Longer explanation
commissioning	buying health services to meet the needs of local people	Commissioning is deciding what healthcare services local people need and buying these. Healthcare services may be bought from various places, for example NHS trusts, private hospitals or voluntary organisations
community health council (CHC)	the patient's watchdog	Community health councils (CHCs) are independent bodies that look after the interests of patients in the NHS. Set up by law, they are sometimes called 'the patient's watchdog'. They keep an eye on the quality of local health services. CHCs have the right to be consulted about major changes to health services in their areas. They also make sure that patients and the public have a fair chance to put forward their views
community health services	healthcare provided outside hospital, in the community	Community health services are provided outside hospital, in the community. They include services provided by district nurses, health visitors and therapists
continuing professional development (CPD)	education and training to keep skills up to date	It is important for all clinical staff (for example nurses, doctors and therapists) to keep their skills up to date. To do this, they need to have 'continuing professional development' – education and training to maintain their skills, and learn new ones

Technical jargon	Short explanation	Longer explanation
controls assurance	a national programme to spot and cut down on risks to NHS organisations	Controls assurance is a national programme to make sure that all NHS organisations: • spot the range of risks facing them. For example, there may be risks in the areas of health and safety, clinical care, managing patients' medical records and staff • cut down on these risks as much as they can. This helps them to provide the best possible care
day case	patient admitted to hospital but not staying overnight	More and more often, you can have an operation, treatment or tests done in one day. If you are admitted to hospital, but do not have to stay the night, you are a 'day case'
Disability Discrimination Act 1995	a law that gives new rights to disabled people	The Disability Discrimination Act 1995 gives new rights to disabled people. These help them find and keep a job, get goods and services, and buy or rent land and property
earned autonomy	more freedom, for doing well	*The NHS Plan* is a government report on making the NHS meet patients' needs better. Under this plan, NHS organisations will be rated using a 'traffic-light' system. Every year, each organisation will be given a red, amber or green light, to show how well it is doing. Those who do well will have more freedom to decide things for themselves. This freedom, for doing well, is called 'earned autonomy'

Technical jargon	Short explanation	Longer explanation
evidence-based healthcare	healthcare that is known to work	It is important that the healthcare we give people works. To be sure that it does, we must keep up to date with good research findings. When healthcare is in keeping with these, we say that it is 'evidence-based'
finished consultant episode (FCE)	a measure of NHS activity	When one consultant has finished caring for a patient, this is called a 'finished consultant episode'. The consultant may discharge the patient or transfer the care of the patient to another consultant
health action zone (HAZ)	scheme that brings together the NHS and other bodies to tackle the causes of ill health in an area	Health action zones bring together the NHS and other bodies to tackle the causes of ill health in an area. They are targeted to areas with poor health, often because of deprivation. By improving people's health, they close the gap between these areas and areas with better health, making things more equal
health authority (HA)	NHS body in charge of improving the health and wellbeing of its local people	Health authorities have the job of improving the health and wellbeing of their local people. Through health improvement programmes (plans about how the health and wellbeing of local people can be improved), they: • make sure that health services for their local people are well planned and provided • improve general health • help reduce gaps in health between people living in different areas

Technical jargon	Short explanation	Longer explanation
health improvement programme (HImP)	a plan for improving the health and wellbeing of local people	With other local organisations and the public, health authorities must come up with a health improvement programme (HImP). This looks at how the health and wellbeing of local people can be improved. The HImP covers five years, three in detail and two in outline
healthy living centre (HLC)	centre funded by lottery money to improve health	The New Opportunities Fund uses lottery money to fund healthy living centres. These centres aim to encourage healthy lifestyles, and so improve health and wellbeing. They try to get public and private sector bodies to work together. Centres may be based in buildings, or may be networks of people working in different parts of the community
inpatient	patient staying overnight in hospital	When you are admitted to hospital and stay overnight, you are an inpatient
inter-agency	linking two or more organisations	As well as the NHS, many other organisations are important to improving health and healthcare, such as social services, housing and education. If something is inter-agency, it involves two or more organisations linking in with each other
intermediate care	care to bridge the gap between hospital and home	Intermediate care helps people who do not need to be in hospital, but are not yet well enough to live at home. It lasts up to six weeks, acting as a bridge between hospital and home. For example, intermediate care can stop older people having to go into a care home

Technical jargon	Short explanation	Longer explanation
Investors in People	an award that shows an organisation is good at training and developing staff	Organisations can apply for the Investors in People award, to show that they are good at training and developing staff. Organisations that get the award must be assessed each year to show that their standards have not slipped
modernisation agenda	the government's plans to improve the NHS	In December 1997, the Labour government published a White Paper (an official report setting out its policy) called *The New NHS: modern, dependable*. This described a ten-year plan for making the NHS more modern, and so improving health and healthcare. The things the NHS must do to make this plan happen are sometimes called the 'modernisation agenda'
multi-agency	involving several organisations	As well as the NHS, many other organisations are important to improving health and healthcare, such as social services, housing and education. If something is multi-agency, it involves several organisations working together
multidisciplinary	involving people from several staff groups	In the NHS, there are many different staff groups. Some are clinical (for example nurses, doctors and therapists), and some are non-clinical (such as managers, porters and medical records staff). If something is multidisciplinary, it involves staff from several different groups working together

Technical jargon	Short explanation	Longer explanation
National Institute for Clinical Excellence (NICE)	the national organisation that tells healthcare staff how best to care for patients	The National Institute for Clinical Excellence provides clinical guidelines. Clinical guidelines tell healthcare staff how best to provide health services. They are based on the results of research, which prove the best way of treating people with different health problems
National Service Framework (NSF)	standards for providing healthcare	National Service Frameworks (NSFs) are standards set out by the government for how the NHS must provide care. They aim to improve quality, and make sure care is equally good everywhere in the country. There are different NSFs for different groups of patients, for example cancer patients, older people and people with diabetes. NSFs are based on the results of research, which prove the best way of treating people with different health problems. They also take into account the views of service users
The NHS Plan: a plan for investment, a plan for reform	a government report on making the NHS meet patients' needs better	The Labour government published *The NHS Plan* in 2000. It follows consultation with healthcare experts, patients, carers and relatives. *The NHS Plan* aims to make the NHS meet patients' needs better. It will also let local NHS organisations decide more things for themselves, if they show they are doing well

Technical jargon	Short explanation	Longer explanation
The New NHS: modern, dependable	a government report on improving the NHS	*The New NHS* is a White Paper (an official report setting out the government's policy), published in 1997. It sets out a ten-year plan for improving the NHS. It aims to make the NHS more modern, and to make sure that people can depend on it to help them when they need it
nicotine replacement therapy (NRT)	a way of helping people to quit smoking	Nicotine replacement therapy helps people to quit or cut down on smoking. It gives them smaller amounts of nicotine in a different way, such as through a skin patch, chewing gum, nose spray or pill. This makes it easier for them to go without cigarettes
nurse consultant	an expert nurse	In the past, nurses who wanted to go further in their careers often had to give up looking after patients and become managers. The job of nurse consultant is a new one. It is aimed at expert nurses who want to go further in their careers, and keep in day-to-day contact with patients. Nurse consultants can provide specialist care to patients
out-of-area treatment (OAT)	one-off treatment not covered by a service agreement	Most NHS treatments and services are covered by service agreements. Service agreements say how much care the provider (organisation providing healthcare) must provide in exchange for an agreed amount of NHS money. Out-of-area treatments are one-off treatments not covered by service agreements, for example if someone gets ill on holiday, away from home

Technical jargon	Short explanation	Longer explanation
outpatient	patient visiting hospital but not being admitted	When you go to hospital for advice or treatment, but are not admitted, you are an outpatient
partnership working	working closely with other people and organisations	In the past, the NHS sometimes worked alone to try to improve health and healthcare. Now, it realises that it needs to work with local people and organisations. For example, there are many 'partner organisations' whose work affects the health of local people. These include local authorities (through housing, education and social services), charities and community groups. Working with partners like these is called 'partnership working'
Patient Advocacy and Liaison Service (PALS)	the new service to help patients who want to complain	By 2002, an NHS-wide Patient Advocacy and Liaison Service (PALS) will be set up in all trusts. Trusts are NHS organisations that provide local healthcare. PALS will help patients who want to complain about trusts' services
personal development plan (PDP)	plan for training and work experience	In the NHS, each member of staff should have a personal development plan. These plans set out what training and work experience the people need to help them do their job better. The plans can also help them to move on to other jobs, if they want to, by getting new skills and experience
primary care	care provided by GPs, dentists, pharmacists or opticians, and their teams	'Primary care' means the first place you go to get health advice or services. This is usually the GP, dentist, pharmacist or optician, and their teams of healthcare staff, such as nurses and therapists

Technical jargon	Short explanation	Longer explanation
primary care group (PCG)	NHS body that brings together GP practices and community nurses	Primary care groups (PCGs) are NHS organisations that bring together GP practices and community nurses. Community nurses are people like district nurses and health visitors. PCGs answer to health authorities (the NHS bodies in charge of improving the health and wellbeing of their local people). There are four levels of PCG. At level one (the basic level), PCGs just advise the health authority. At level four, they are free-standing bodies, known as 'primary care trusts'
primary care trust (PCTs)	free-standing NHS body that brings together GP practices and community nurses	There are four levels of primary care group (PCG), the NHS bodies that bring together GP practices and community nurses. At level four (the highest level), PCGs are free-standing bodies, known as 'primary care trusts' (PCTs). PCTs buy health services to meet the needs of their local people, and also provide community health services (healthcare outside hospital, in the community)

Technical jargon	Short explanation	Longer explanation
private finance initiative (PFI)	a system for getting private companies to help with NHS projects	The government is encouraging the public and private sectors to work together in partnership. The private finance initiative (PFI) is one type of 'Public Private Partnership' (PPP). PFI aims to improve quality and value for money in the NHS. It gets private sector companies to invest money in NHS projects, and to help out where they have useful skills. For example, if an NHS hospital needs a new building, it may look for a private sector partner to design, build and pay for this. The private sector company may also run some non-clinical services, such as cleaning and maintaining the building. PFI is designed to benefit both the NHS and the private partner
provider	body that provides health-care	Providers are the bodies that provide healthcare. They may be NHS or private bodies. For example, providers include trusts, GP practices and private hospitals
Saving Lives: our healthier nation	a government report on improving health	*Saving Lives* is a White Paper (an official report setting out the government's policy), published in 1999. It sets out the government's plans for improving health. *Saving Lives* focuses on heart disease and stroke, accidents, cancer and mental health. It includes targets for cutting the numbers of deaths from these health problems

Technical jargon	Short explanation	Longer explanation
secondary care	hospital care	'Secondary care' is care that you are referred to by a health professional in primary care. This could be your GP, dentist or optician, or one of their team of healthcare staff, such as a nurse or therapist. Secondary care is usually provided at a hospital. For example, your GP might send you to see a hospital consultant about a health problem
Single Regeneration Budget (SRB)	money to help local partnerships put new life into their area	The Single Regeneration Budget (SRB) is money to help local people and organisations work together to put new life into their area. It is available to areas with severe need, and is used to help get the community involved and to get business going. The government sees the SRB as important in making things more equal between different areas in England
stakeholder	someone with an interest in health services	Stakeholders are people or organisations that have an interest in health and healthcare, such as members of the public and community groups. The NHS is expected to involve stakeholders in making plans and deciding things. For example, stakeholders may be asked to give their views on how good local healthcare is, and on any plans to change services

Technical jargon	Short explanation	Longer explanation
standardised mortality ratio (SMR)	a measure of death rates	Standardised mortality ratios (SMRs) compare death rates in a given area with those in England and Wales as a whole. SMRs take into account the different ages of the people compared. An SMR of 100 is average. A higher number means there is a higher death rate than you would expect, and a lower one a lower death rate. For example, an SMR of 150 shows the death rate is 50% above the national average. An SMR of 70 shows the death rate is 30% below the national average
Sure Start	a scheme to help young children in deprived areas	Sure Start aims to give better chances to children in deprived areas. It aims to make sure that all children are ready to learn when they get to school. Sure Start is aimed at children under 4 years old. It involves the NHS and local government working together
tertiary care	very specialist care, for rare or complex health problems	'Tertiary care' is care you are referred to by a health professional in secondary (hospital) care, usually a hospital consultant. Tertiary care is very specialist, for rare or complex health problems
triage	a system of sorting people into groups, based on how ill they are	The word 'triage' was first used in the army, in wartime. It means sorting the wounded into three groups, based on how badly injured they are. Accident and emergency (casualty) departments now use triage. This helps them make sure that they treat the people with the most urgent health problems first. They may sort people into three groups, or often more

Technical jargon	Short explanation	Longer explanation
trust	an NHS organisation that provides local healthcare	NHS trusts are the organisations that provide local healthcare. They may provide a number of types of care, such as hospital, community, mental health or ambulance services
to vire	to move funds from one budget to another	In the NHS, an organisation's funding is split into different budgets. Each budget covers different costs, for example services, staffing or drugs. Sometimes an organisation might decide to move funds from one budget to another. For example, they might be running short of money in one area but have more in another. This is called 'viring' or 'virement'

EXAMPLE OF A SHORT STYLE GUIDE

> **Note**
>
> This is an example of an in-house style guide, based on one I produced for a health authority. It does not cover all eight of the guidelines exactly as set out in Chapter 7. This is because it was designed to fit the particular organisation's needs and preferences. If you decide to write your own short style guide like this, you can tailor it precisely to your organisation, staff and typical target audience.

GENERAL

1 Make use of the spell check, grammar check and thesaurus facilities on your computer.

PLAIN ENGLISH

2 Aim for an average sentence length of 15–20 words, but with some variation.
3 Avoid words that do not add to the message.

Before: 'Many of the functions sketched out for health authority action are around playing a key role in...'
After: 'Health authorities have a key role in...'

4   Avoid foreign words.

    Before: 'The Health Authority's position vis-à-vis capitation target...'
    After: 'The Health Authority's position on its capitation target...'

5   Avoid unusual words.

    Before: 'The paucity of qualified staff...'
    After: 'The shortage of qualified staff...'

6   Use active verbs.

    Before: 'Meetings have been held by the Health Authority...'
    After: 'The Health Authority has held meetings...'

7   Use verbs rather than abstract nouns.

    Before: 'There is agreement across all organisations.'
    After: 'All organisations agree.'
    Before: 'We are not alone in carrying out a review of services.'
    After: 'We are not alone in reviewing services.'

8   Avoid cross-references to other documents that are not freely available
    to likely readers.
9   Use lists that are bullet-pointed (using a plain, round bullet) or, where it
    enhances meaning, numbered (using roman numerals, to avoid confu-
    sion with section numbers). Leave a line between each bullet point and
    put a full stop at the end of the list.

    Before: '...the overall benefits of proposals in terms of the right clinical
    quality; the fair distribution of, and access to, services; and improved
    effectiveness and efficiency of individual treatments and services as a
    whole.'
    After: '...the overall benefits of proposals in terms of:

    *   the right clinical quality
    *   the fair distribution of, and access to, services
    *   improved effectiveness and efficiency of:
        – individual treatments
        – services as a whole.'

ABBREVIATIONS AND ACRONYMS

10 At the first mention within the text (i.e. not in titles), always write the
    words out fully and put the abbreviation or acronym in brackets. After
    that, just use the abbreviation or acronym.

NUMBERS IN TEXT

11 The basic rule is that in text, numbers from one to ten are expressed as words, and numbers 11 and above as figures.

12 But express in words any number that begins a sentence.

Example: 'Thirty patients...'

13 And express as figures:

- dates, times, measurements, percentages and values

Examples: '11 June', '9.30 a.m.', '5 miles', '6 per cent' (in text), '6%' (in tables), '£1.2 million', '£4,700'

- numbers following nouns such as 'page', 'chapter', 'section', etc.

Examples: 'page 2', 'section 5', 'clause 1.3'

14 In lists of numbers, do not mix words or figures; use one or the other, depending on whether more of them are above or below 11.

Examples:
- 'Two, four and twenty-five...'
- '8, 11 and 23...'

15 Use commas to mark numbers of 1,000 or more into groups of three, from the right.

Examples:
- '22,543' (rather than '22543')
- '12,500,650' (rather than '12500650')

EQUALITY IN WRITING

16 Views vary on how acceptable it is to use male pronouns ('he', 'him', etc.) to refer to men and women. Even if you think it is fine to do so, some readers will not, so it makes sense to avoid detracting from your message by using male terms.

17 Using 'his/her' or 'his or her', etc. as an alternative can sound clumsy, and can often be avoided by using the plural or by simple rephrasing.

Before: 'Payments to individual board or other PCG members must be approved by the PCG chair in his/her capacity as PCG responsible officer.'

After: (using the plural) 'Payments to individual board or other PCG members must be approved by the PCG chairs in their capacity as PCG responsible officers.'

After: (rephrasing) 'As PCG responsible officer, the PCG chair must approve payments to individual board or other PCG members...'

18   When referring to people, be consistent in the form of address.

Before: (in a list of Primary Care Group Board members) 'Dr J O'Riley, Dr E Farnsworth, Dr D Regan, Gillian Smith, Rachel Chatsworth, Pam Jones, Peter Harrison, Ralph Briggs...'

After: 'Dr John O'Riley, Dr Eric Farnsworth, Dr David Regan, Ms Gillian Smith, Mrs Rachel Chatsworth, Miss Pam Jones, Mr Peter Harrison, Mr Ralph Briggs...'

(or 'John O'Riley, Eric Farnsworth, David Regan, Gillian Smith, Rachel Chatsworth, Pam Jones, Peter Harrison, Ralph Briggs...')

19   In some non-European names, the first name and surname may be reversed. If in doubt, ask for clarification.

APOSTROPHES

20   When using apostrophes to show ownership, put the apostrophe before the 's' when the owner is singular.

Examples: 'the Health Authority's strategy', 'the nurse's contract'

21   This includes collective nouns, where the noun is singular but refers to more than one person or thing.

Examples: 'the staff's responsibilities', 'the committee's decision'

22   'Its', meaning 'belonging to it', does not take an apostrophe. The only use of 'it's' is as a shortened form of 'it is' (and would not therefore be used in formal writing).

Example: 'The Health Authority will make its decision...'

23   When the owner is plural, put the apostrophe after the 's'.

Examples: 'the GPs' premises', 'the members' forum'

24   However, where the noun is already plural before the 's' is added, put the apostrophe before the 's'.

    Examples: 'women's services', 'children's rights'

25   If the owner's name ends in 's', go with how you would say it. Add an apostrophe and another 's' if you would pronounce the second 's'; do not if you would not.

    Examples: 'Fiona Divers' computer', 'Chris's desk'

26   The plural of abbreviations does not take an apostrophe unless you are expressing ownership.

    Examples:
    (no ownership expressed) 'The GPs have agreed that. . .'
    (ownership expressed) 'We have noted the GPs' agreement. . .'

CAPITALISATION

27   Use capitals for all NHS organisations, in line with national guidance.

    Examples:
    'NHS Executive', 'Health Authorities', 'NHS Trusts'

    (**Note:** Most published style guides advise that it looks better and is more sensible to use small letters when writing about NHS organisations in general, and capitals for specific organisations. For example, you would say 'Primary care groups are responsible for. . .' but 'Wilmington Primary Care Group (*or* 'the Primary Care Group') is responsible for. . .' However, in 1999, the NHS Executive sent out a memo saying that initial capital letters should be used for writing about NHS organisations in general. The Health Authority felt it should follow this guidance, although I have since seen many NHS documents that do not. I suspect many people never realised they should be doing so.)

28   Do not use capital letters for:

    ●   Medical conditions (unless part of the term is a person's name)

    Examples: 'diabetes', 'cancer', 'coronary heart disease', 'Down's syndrome'

- Specialties and professions (unless used to refer to a particular department, directorate, etc.)

Examples: 'orthopaedics', 'midwifery' (but 'X-Ray at Wilmington Hospital has seen 2,654 patients...')

- Positions (except when referring to specific people)

Examples: 'NHS Trust chairs' (but 'the Health Authority Chair...')

- Concepts

Examples: 'clinical governance', 'quality', 'lifelong learning'

INDEX

abbreviations 6
  explaining 79–80
  style guide example 154
abstract nouns 7, 69–70
academic writing 33
accommodation 35–6
acronyms 6
  explaining 79–80
  style guide example 154
active verbs 70–2
activities 6
Acts of Parliament 5
agreeing explanations of technical
    jargon 80
aids to jargon busting
  buzz words translations 115–19
  gobbledegook translations 121–34
  technical jargon explanations 135–51
'and', beginning sentences with 33, 68
Anglo-Saxon words 66
apostrophes
  style guide example 156–7
approaches 6
attitudes, inappropriate 31–2
Australia 24

bafflegab see gobbledegook
barriers see plain language: barriers
bed, definition 6
behaviour change
  features likely to lead to 41

blind people 109–10
bodies 5
bold fonts 58
Braille transcriptions 109
budgets 6
bullet points for lists 68–9
bureaucratese see gobbledegook
'but', beginning sentences with 33, 68
buzz words 4–5, 8
  characteristics 11
  clichés 8, 12
  obscurity of meaning 12
  in speech 106
  sports jargon in management 9
  tackling 76
    examples 82–9
    summary flowchart 81
  teamwork images 9
  from technical jargon of other areas
      of life 8–9
  translations 115–19

Canada 24
capitals, use in documents 58
  style guide example 157–8
care types and services 5
categorising jargon see recognising and
    categorising jargon
change management skills 19
clearer thinking 28–9
clichés 8, 12

clinical conditions 5
clinical governance 10
clinical specialities 5
clinical treatments 5
colleagues' comments, testing
  documents 98
colour in documents 59
communications, definition viii
complex structures 7
concepts 6
condescending, plain language seen as
  34–5
consultants 19, 20
  testing documents 98–9
convincing people 31—9
courses 20, 21

deaf people 110
design
  documents 56–7, 57–9
  electronic media communication
    107–8
deverbal nouns 69
diagnoses, medical terms for 12
documents
  definition viii
  legal 24, 34
  planning
    bold fonts 58
    capitals 58
    colour 59
    design 56–7, 57–9
    emphasis 58
    font style and size 57
    guidelines, not rules 52
    in-house production 56
    italic fonts 58
    justification 58
    layout 56–7, 57–9
    left-aligned text 58
    paper weight and finish 58
    plain language elements 51–2
    right-aligned text 58
    setting the brief 54–5
    structuring documents 55–6
    target audience, importance 52–3

    templates 59
    underlined text 58
    white space 58
    word-processing software 59
  process 105
  revising see testing and revising below
  technical jargon 5
  testing and revising
    areas to test 91
    choosing methods 101–2
    colleagues' comments 98
    consultants 98–9
    methods of testing 92–100
    plain English experts 98–9
    readability formulae 93–8
    real audience testing 99–100
    self-checking 93
    text-editing software 93–8
doublespeak see gobbledegook

electronic media communication 107–8
elements of plain language 51–2
emphasis in documents 58
equality in writing 63–4
  style guide example 155–6
ethnic minorities 111–12
European Union 24
evidence
  sources 23–5
    negative jargon use 36
  surveys 37
examples
  buzz words translations 115–19
  gobbledegook 7–8
    translations 121–34
  style guide 153–8
  tackling NHS jargon 82–9
  technical jargon explanations 135–51
explaining technical jargon see technical
  jargon

familiar words and phrases 65–7
feedback 46–7
first person, writing in 72
Flesch-Kincaid Grade Level readability
  formula 93, 94

Flesch Reading Ease scores 96, *97*
FOG *see* gobbledegook
font style and size *57*
foreign words 7, 66
forms 24–5
funds *6*

glossaries
   comprehensive, for use of whole
      organisation 80
   providing in documents 79
gobbledegook 4, 6–7
   abstract nouns 7
   characteristics *11*
   complex structures 7
   examples 7–8
   foreign words 7
   impersonal tone 7
   long sentences 7
   long words 7
   plain English alternatives 12
   in speech 7, 106
   tackling 77
      examples 82–9
      summary flowchart 81
   translations 121–34
   unusual words 7
government action *24*
grammar 32–3, 61–3
grammar checkers 62
   readability formulae 93–7
graphic designers 56
guidelines to plain language *see* plain
   language: guidelines
Gunning Fog Index 93, *94–6*

habit, plain language barrier 36–7
hard of hearing, people who are 110
house style 43

impersonal tone of gobbledegook 7
in-house production of documents 56
information design 51
initiatives *6*
innocent reasons for negative jargon use
   32–3

internal communications
   plain language benefits 25
involving people 41–7
italic fonts *58*

jargon, definition 4
justification, text *58*

kitemarking 98
knowledge, plain language facts 19

Latin words 66
law 24
layout
   documents 56–7, *57–9*
   electronic media communication
      107–8
left-aligned text *58*
legal documents 24, 34
length of sentences 68–9
lists, bullet points for 68–9
long sentences 7, 97
long words 7, 97
longer words 65–6

management commitment 39
managers' needs 47
measures *6*
medical terms for diagnoses 12
Microsoft Word grammar checker 93, 96
misspellings 63
misunderstanding terms 77–8
money
   requirements 18–19
   savings 25, *26*, 27

negative jargon use 12
   evidence sources *36*
   innocent reasons for 32–3
negative statements 72–3
New Zealand *24*
NHS communicators, definition vii-viii
NHS Identity Guidelines 56–7
nouns
   abstract 7, 69–70
   deverbal 69

numbers in text
  style guide example 155

obscurity of meaning of buzz words 12
official names *see* technical jargon
officialese *see* gobbledegook
Old English words 66
older people 110
ordinary words used as technical jargon
  6

paper weight and finish *58*
partially sighted people 109–10
passive verbs 70–2
patients
  care improvements 25
  relations improvements 25, 27–8
phrases, plain *see* writing plainly: plain
  words and phrases
plain-communicating organisations 17
  benefits, describing to staff 23–9
  convincing people 31–9
  implementing plain language 18
  involving people, linking research to
    practice 41–7
  money requirements 18–19
  research evidence, putting into
    practice *18*
  resources required 18–21
  time requirements 18–19
  training 20, *21*
plain English alternatives to
  gobbledegook 12
Plain English Campaign *19*
Plain English Commission *20*
plain language 12
  barriers
    attitudes, inappropriate 31–2
    condescending, plain language seen
      as 34–5
    habit 36–7
    implementing, too much trouble for
      too little reward 38
    perceptions of 'proper' English 32–3
    simplistic, plain language seen as
      34

using jargon to fit in 35–6
    values, inappropriate 31–2
  benefits
    clearer thinking 28–9
    internal communications 25
    money savings 25, *26*, 27
    patient care improvements 25
    patient relations improvements 25,
      27–8
    public relations improvements 25,
      27–8
    staff relations improvements 27–8
    time savings 25, *26*
    wanted by staff 25
    written communications, based on
      24
  condescending, seen as 34–5
  consultants *see* consultants
  convincing people 39
  elements 51–2
  evidence sources 23–5
  feedback 46–7
  guidelines
    blind people 109–10
    deaf people 110
    document planning 51–9
    electronic media communication
      107–8
    ethnic minorities 111–12
    hard of hearing, people who are
      110
    jargon, tackling 75–89
    older people 110
    partially sighted people 109–10
    reading difficulties, people with
      110–11
    skills in understanding and
      applying 19
    special needs audiences 109–12
    speech communications 103–7
    style guides 43
    testing and revising documents 91–
      102
    writing difficulties, people with
      110–11
    writing plainly 61–73

implementing 18
    too much trouble for too little
        reward 38
    involving everyone 47
    knowledge of facts 19
    management commitment 39
    reading faster *27–8*
    reference books on plain English *53–4*
    resources 53–4
    simplistic, seen as 34
    skills 19
    style guides 42–6
    training 42
    understanding better *27–8*
    worldwide movements *24*
Plain Language International Network
    24
plain phrases *see* writing plainly: plain
    words and phrases
plain sentences *see* writing plainly
plain words and phrases *see* writing
    plainly
planned speech 104, *105*
planning
    documents *see* documents
    speech communications 104
political correctness 63
    style guide example 155–6
political writing 32
positive jargon use 12
positive statements *72–3*
posts 5
prepositions 33
printers 56
processes *6*
professionals, use of jargon 31–2
programmes 6
'proper' English, perceptions of 32–3
public relations improvements 25,
    27–8
published style guides, examples *43–4*
punctuation 63

readability formulae 93–8
reading difficulties, people with 110–11
reading faster *27–8*

real audience testing of documents 99–
    100
recognising and categorising jargon
    3–4
    buzz words 8–9
    characteristics of NHS jargon *11*
    gobbledegook 6–8
    mixed jargon types 9
    technical jargon 5–6
    types of jargon 4–5
    value of jargon 9–12
reference books
    blind or partially sighted people *109*
    electronic media communication *108*
    equality in writing *64*
    grammar *62*
    older people *110*
    plain English *53–4*
    punctuation *63*
    reading difficulties, people with *111*
    style guides *43–4*
    writing difficulties, people with *111*
repeating words 67–8
research
    evidence, putting into practice *18*
    practice, linking to 41–7
resources
    plain language 53–4
    required 18–21
revising documents *see* documents:
        testing and revising
right-aligned text *58*
Romance words 66

second person, writing in 72
self-checking documents 93
sentences, plain *see* writing plainly:
        plain sentences
setting the brief, document planning
    54–5
shop talk *see* technical jargon
short phrases 65–7
short sentences 97
short words 65–7, 97
skills
    change management 19

plain language 19
  training organisations *19–20*
South Africa *24*
special needs audiences 109–12
speech
  buzz words 106
  communications 103–4
    planning 104
    speaking plainly 106
    testing and revising 107
  gobbledegook 7, 106
  planned 104, *105*
  spontaneous 7, 104, *105*
  technical jargon 106
spell checkers 63
spelling 63
split infinitives 32
spontaneous speech 7, 104, *105*
sports jargon in management 9
staff
  benefits to, describing 23–9
  groups 5
  relations improvements 27–8
standards 6
Statutes 5
stripetrouser *see* gobbledegook
structure
  documents 55–6
  electronic media communication *107*
style guides 42
  advantages 44
  areas included *42–3*
  disadvantages 44
  example 153–8
  house style 43
  limitations and solutions 45–6
  plain language guidelines 43
  published, examples *43–4*
Stylewriter-the Plain English Editor 62
surveys *37*
Sweden *24*

tape recording of written text 109
target audience, importance 52–3
teamwork images 9

technical jargon 4
  acronyms and abbreviations 6
  as buzz words of other areas of life
    8–9
  categories 5–6
  characteristics *11*
  explaining 10
    acronyms and abbreviations 79–80
    agreeing explanations 80
    deciding what to explain 77–8
    examples 82–9
    glossaries, providing 79
    methods 78–9
    re-explaining 79
    in speech 106
    summary flowchart 81
  explanations 135–51
  glossaries
    comprehensive, for use of whole
      organisation 80
    providing in documents 79
  medical terms for diagnoses 12
  necessity for 9
  ordinary words used as 6
  in speech 106
  unfamiliarity with 9–10
  usefulness of 9
  value of 9–12
templates, documents 59
testing and revising
  documents *see* documents
  speech communications 107
text-editing software, testing documents
    93–8
texts, definition viii
thesauruses 66
thinking, clearer 28–9
Tim Albert Training *20*
time
  requirements 18–19
  savings 25, *26*
training 20, *21*
  organisations *19–20*
  plain language 42
  templates, location and use 59

underlined text *58*
understanding better *27–8*
unfamiliarity with technical jargon
    9–10
United States *24*
unusual words *7*
usefulness of technical jargon *9*
useless words and phrases *65*

value of technical jargon *9–12*
values, inappropriate *31–2*
verbs
    active *70–2*
    passive *70–2*
    use rather than abstract nouns *69–70*

white space in documents *58*
The Word Centre *20*
word-processing software *59*
    grammar checkers *62, 93*
    spell checkers *63*
words, plain *see* writing plainly: plain
    words and phrases
worldwide movements
    plain language *24*
writing difficulties, people with *110–11*
writing plainly
    equality *63–4*
        style guide example *155–6*

grammar *61–3*
    plain language guidelines *64*
    plain phrases *see* plain words and
        phrases *below*
    plain sentences *64*
        active rather than passive verbs
            70–2
        bullet points for lists *68–9*
        first and second person *72*
        length *68–9*
        positive rather than negative
            statements *72–3*
        verbs rather than abstract nouns
            69–70
    plain words and phrases *64*
        foreign words *66*
        longer words *65–6*
        repeating words *67–8*
        short, familiar words and phrases
            65–7
        thesauruses *66*
        useless words and phrases *65*
    political correctness *63*
        style guide example *155–6*
    punctuation *63*
    spelling *63*
    or translating jargon *75–6*
written communications, benefits based
    on *24*